# HOME WORKOUT

Best Home Exercises for Your Body Fitness and
Strength Training

(Loose Weight Easily Without Leaving Your Home)

## Gloria Caudill

Published by Andrew Zen

# Gloria Caudill

All Rights Reserved

*Home Workout: Best Home Exercises for Your Body Fitness and Strength Training (Loose Weight Easily Without Leaving Your Home)*

ISBN 978-1-77485-198-2

All rights reserved. No part of this guide may be reproduced in any form without permission in writing from the publisher except in the case of brief quotations embodied in critical articles or reviews.

Legal & Disclaimer

The information contained in this book is not designed to replace or take the place of any form of medicine or professional medical advice. The information in this book has been provided for educational and entertainment purposes only.

The information contained in this book has been compiled from sources deemed reliable, and it is accurate to the best of the Author's knowledge; however, the Author cannot guarantee its accuracy and validity and cannot be held liable for any errors or omissions. Changes are periodically made to this book. You must consult your doctor or get professional medical advice before using any of the suggested remedies, techniques, or information in this book.

Upon using the information contained in this book, you agree to hold harmless the Author from and against any damages, costs, and expenses, including any legal fees potentially resulting from the application of any of the information provided by this guide. This disclaimer applies to any damages or injury caused by the use and application, whether directly or indirectly, of any advice or information presented, whether for breach of contract, tort, negligence, personal injury, criminal intent, or under any other cause of action.

You agree to accept all risks of using the information presented inside this book. You need to consult a professional medical practitioner in order to ensure you are both able and healthy enough to participate in this program.

# Table of Contents

# Introduction

Do you desire to have a the strength and flexibility of your body and increase your endurance? There is no need to join a fitness center to attain this. In the comfort at home you can do exercises to improve your body's condition and strengthen your muscles. The simple exercises are done using something a lot simpler and unique resistance bands.

This portable lightweight device can provide advantages that you might not expect from a basic device.

The story of the fitness band dates far back and the enduring nature of its usage proves its efficiency as a fitness device. It's not as classic as traditional weights, however its novelty and effectiveness of the resistance band make them distinctive. The original prototype of resistance bands was created in 1895. We can see it as a contemporary invention. It was developed for gymnastics training because it is a tool for improving the flexibility. When people tried it, they realized that resistance bands can also enhance other physical capacities, such as the endurance and strength.

If you're a fitness fanatic with access to higher-end equipment then why would you not make use of a simple easy resistance band?

In the 1960s Resistance bands became popular in the 1960's. They were used in physical therapy. The therapists and doctors made use of the rehabilitation effects of exercises using resistance bands on muscles, resulting in the strength and flexibility.

After two decades, after the fitness revolution the resistance band finally became an excellent exercise tool. It was popular with the public and the production was at a highest.

These days, resistance bands compete with traditional weights when it comes to increasing the physique of a person. The book you'll discover the advantages and benefits that resistance bands provide to your well-being. This book will also provide the most important and effective exercises. Within a couple of weeks, you'll know that your investment in effort, time and or effort on a band you choose will reap benefits that are far beyond your expectations.

# Chapter 1: Why You Want To Workout At Home And Warming Up

The majority of people admit that it's difficult to maintain a regular workout routine because of obligations to family as well as friends and work. And then there's the task to keep your house tidy and making sure that you are well-prepared for the next week. This book is a great solution for people who can't afford a gym or don't live near the gym.

Whatever the reason, you'd prefer working at home, you would like your time at the gym being the main thing for you. Don't let anyone take your time away and you shouldn't feel guilty for spending a bit of time or money into your workout at home.

While there are a lot of activities in the book in which you can build your own equipment, or do not use it of it, the amount you invest in it must feel like you're paying for your happiness. It's not just about having an exercise routine you can adhere to help you look great however, you'll be feeling much better psychologically. Stress and tension can hide in our brains and muscles. We must work our muscles to eliminate tension and stress. You will never regret getting stronger.

The author of this book is aiming to help you develop an exercise routine you can adhere to since you can complete it at your home. It is essential to create the space at home that you are at ease within. It is crucial to eliminate any distractions in this space as much as you can and that includes locking out pets and If you have kids take them to a caregiver or entertain them. This workout at home is likely be your getaway as well as your time to relax.

For many, putting an effective workout playlist is essential to get the most benefit from it. The right music can inspire your body, allow you to accelerate your progress, and boost the amount of adrenaline you release. You can find playlists made via the Internet or through radio apps. It is important to keep in mind is that headphones that have a cord can block your path and the Bluetooth inside your ear will be sweaty. A Bluetooth wireless speaker with a built-in microphone is suggested. The most well-known music genre is hip-hop due to the bass line, however depending on your preferences, it could sound like classical that keeps you moving. It is important to personalize your schedule to suit you since it's one of the best things you do for yourself throughout the day.

Sort out your workout clothes. Do whatever you can to get rid of any excuses that have held you back from achieving your goals before. Even if you're changing from a fitness enthusiast to exercising at home, staying as organized with your homework can lead to success and you will never regret this choice.

This book you'll learn how investing in some items to start will make a big impact. The first item that is suggested to perform these exercises is barbells. A barbell is a straightforward piece of equipment that can be utilized in many ways, as you'll discover. is an entire chapter dedicated to the barbell routine.

The second piece of equipment to consider is the dumbbells. There's also a section that is dedicated solely to dumbbell exercises. They are also able to provide a variety of exercises for strengthening and cutting fat. Both dumbbells and barbells are able to be used to build endurance and also for aerobic workouts while trimming fat off of the body.

An essential step to stick to a schedule is to prepare your mind to face the obstacles. It's helpful to picture you are doing your routine prior to you begin. Be sure that all the equipment you will need to plan your routine is set to start. Keep track of your workouts in order to monitor your performance. You will be able to see which weights you have graduated from and the way you've improved the repetitions. It is a great motivator to see the figures.

Another trick to keep you motivated is to document your progress on photos. Keep a photo journal of your beginning body as well as the body you're currently working on. These pictures will help you see how far you've come and help you keep going.

Most people will keep your routine private when you're just starting out could be the most effective way to go. It is best to allow people to be aware of how you've changed. However, for certain people, they might want to find someone to partner during the home workout to help them be accountable. Whatever you chooseto do, stick to your plan. Nobody else can make this happen for you, only you. If you're feeling like giving up Try to remember why you decided to do it.

Keep in mind that the fact that you have a goal to accomplish is something that should be a source of pride. It's your choice how you arrange your timetable to be able to accommodate the new, healthier you. If you're well-behaved and are transitioning from an exercise facility to a at-home workout, you can take pride in the time and money you'll benefit by not visiting an expensive gym.

Home Workout Pros and Cons

Pros:

1.) Your personal space 1. Personal Space. If the thought of going for a workout makes you feel anxious or self-conscious, a house exercise will keep everyone from who is watching you while you sweat. This allows you to experiment with new workout techniques or routines without fear of what people will consider or observe.

2.) Time saver 2) Time Saver: You'll save tons of time without having to carry your gym bag, go by car or on foot into the fitness center. You will be able to make use of all your exercise by using the extra time you'd be spending traveling. it will reduce the excuses you have to stay away from working out.

3.) Saving Money: Get the most of your earnings and perform your exercise at home instead of paying for gym memberships each month. This will guarantee that, if the financial circumstances change you won't be unable to exercise due to the expense of gym membership.

4.) Improve your workout You don't need to think about people who are around you, you will be able to concentrate on your training. You'll be less distracted and develop the ability to be your own personal trainer.

Cons:

1.) Concentrating: Make sure that if not live on your own You establish boundaries with your roommate and family members. They should be aware that this is important to you and why you should be completely alone. You will also be able to switch off your mobile phone, and not have the television or computer within your fitness space.

2.) buying some equipment 2) Buying Some Gear: You can decide to invest either a tiny or a large amount into your fitness routine at home or do absolutely nothing. This is the reason we have written this book to show how you can perform exercises using your body weight as equipment. We've even provided examples of how you can use your household items to make weights, or even your broom as a barbell. There are no excuses.

It is evident that the benefits outweigh the negatives. This is the reason you are currently reading this. It is sensible to do this from your home, in privacy and save cash.

Let's get started. The most important aspect of any exercise regardless of what form you're in, will be your warm-up phase. It can prevent injuries and increase your results. Your muscles will appreciate it.

Warming Up

There are numerous benefits for consistently warming up prior to doing a weight-training workout. The people who consistently perform exercises that require weights place lots of stress upon their joint.

Joint injuries are quite frequent among weightlifters who are serious. Remember this when you train, you should prepare properly prior to your workouts in order to avoid these types of injuries by bringing your blood circulation as well as increasing oxygen levels in your body prior to performing the exercises to build strength.

The way you start your workout is the choice you make, there are a variety of suggestions to are followed, but that's the beauty of designing your own home workout to suit your individual requirements and schedule.

Benefits of Warming Up

* Increases the temperature of muscles Speed and flexibility increase.

* The body temperature is elevated prevents muscle strain

Dilated Blood Vessels: Increase blood flow and reduce tension

* Improved mental focus

* Improved recovery after finishing with the exercise

Easy Ways to Warm Up

Do not repeat repetition of the same routine each when you are warming up to prevent your body from becoming accustomed to it.

You might want to focus on the areas of your body you've identified during your exercise

* Cardio that is quick and incorporated with stretching works best

* Run through your drive for 10 mins, then sprint for 1 minute, then stop or walk back to the same spot and repeat

* Bike through the neighborhood, speeding up at times

* Ten minutes of jump rope

* Brisk walk around the block or in your yard a few times

* Dancing to the beat for 10 minutes

Stretching

The necessity to stretch prior to exercising can affect your endurance and flexibility overall. It is strongly suggested prior to and after your workouts.

In general the stretching process improves oxygen circulation and blood flow across the entire body. This helps prepare your muscles for a weight-training routine.

Additionally, if done often, stretching can improve your joint flexibility as well as relieve tension in your muscles. It will allow you to unwind after your workout, making it easier to sleep at night, which can improve your workouts as well as your daily life.

Benefits of Stretching

* Expand your flexibility

Improve blood circulation

* Release tension in muscles

* Increases levels of normal hormones and reduces stress reactions

* Energy boosts

Simple and Beneficial Stretches

Bear Crawl

This is a great move to stretch and warm up. You'll want to bend your knees and place your hands behind yourself on the floor. Do not do this in socks. You will require a grip to avoid falling and inflicting an injury. Make yourself crouch to a bear-like posture and then begin using your hands and feet to walk as the bear for one minute at a stretch, then repeat for five minutes. It will stretch all your muscles and, over time, you'll become more proficient at doing it.

Hamstring

As you sit down, place your left leg in front of your and then bend your left knee. Try to get your toes to touch. Do this for 15 to

20 minutes. Then, switch to stretching the right leg.

Calf Muscle Stretch

Place your feet on the wall. Set your left foot behind you by about a foot and set it on the floor , without benting your knee. Set your hands on the wall and then bend the right knee in order to stretch the left calves. Keep it for about 15 minutes. Change to putting your left foot behind your right and repeat the steps for this leg.

Lower Back Stretch

Do this by lying on the floor flat, with your back to towards the ceiling. It is recommended to bring your knees toward your chest. Take your knees by your hands and push them towards the upper part the body. Then, lift your shoulders a bit to get maximum stretch. Try moving your body back and forth small amount. You'll be able to feel it and feel the tension disappearing from your body. Do this for 30 minutes.

## Quad Stretch

Begin by lying onto the back of your physique with the right knee bent to the knee. Lift your left leg toward your chest, then grab your left ankle with your left hand. Then, pull your left ankle towards to the center of your back. Maintain the position for twenty minutes. Then switch to stretching the left side quads.

## Good Mornings

Put your hands behind your head creating wings with your elbows. Hold your hips in a hinge and gently bend your knees. While doing this, allow your core muscles bend towards the front. Concentrate on your core and work your core muscles. For a short time, hold the position, then move your hips back, lift your core, then get up to a standing position. Repeat the Good Mornings for one minute.

## Half Moon Twists

Place your body on your back flat. Place one knee on your stomach. Cradle it with the opposite hand. Then gently pull that knee over your body and towards the floor. Make sure that both shoulder blades firmly on the ground. Your aim is to stretch your spine and squeeze your organs. Make sure to get your knee to the floor If you can't achieve that, don't be concerned if your knee can not get all the way towards the ground. If you feel a little resistance within your lower back quit trying to go further. There will be a deep stretch through your legs. Do this for five breaths. Repeat on the other side.

The More You Know About Stretching, the Better

The aging process and your exercise routine can impact your flexibility. It is crucial that following an exercise, you have enough time to stretch to stretch again. By doing this it will help your muscles retain their flexibility, but they'll become stronger. A program of exercise that incorporates the three components (cardiovascular strength, strength and flexibility) will help keep your tendons and muscles in the best condition possible.

Stretching Burns Fat

Although stretching makes you more flexible, it also can help you burn calories and relax after a strenuous exercise. The act of stretching can reduce blood pressure after a strenuous exercise.

It is recommended to stretch all muscles, instead of just the ones that focus on the weak spots in your body. Your muscles work together, and if you leave one area out of stretching and stretch, you will not achieve the maximum benefit from the stretching.

It is something that we do in our daily lives. You move your toes around in order to stretch, and lift your arms and bend your back when exhausted. These movements are actually stretching exercises; you must just go further before you begin an exercise routine.

It is not a requirement for the most amount of amount of time for stretching. Stretching can be done in one to fifteen minutes or less It is easy to incorporate into your exercise routine.

Apart from the benefits of being prepared and reducing your chance of getting injured in a workout Here are some additional reasons to make stretching an important part of your routine.

Increases Your Optimism

Intentionally putting on too much tension in your body can create a myriad of problems, such as stress and tension. The stretching process releases the good chemicals in your brain , leaving you feeling calmer and at ease. When you go to bed at night it is a great practice to make you feel more relaxed when you lie down, leading to an improved night's rest and a more positive start to the day.

Improves Your Posture

Through stretching that stretch your muscles, you can relax and lengthen muscles that have become tight and are pushing your body into the incorrect direction creating discomfort and poor posture.

Increased Flexibility

The most obvious change to the body following stretching is flexibility mobility, mobility, and flexibility. A great workout routine should include stretching, without a doubt to decrease the chance of injury.

Increase in Endurance

Stretching muscles relaxes them and boosts blood flow. The more you exercise and get tired, the more exhausted your muscles become which can cause you to become mentally exhausted.

Decreases Risk of Injury

It can help provide an increased supply of nutrients to muscles, which will reduce muscle soreness and speeding the recovery process from joint and muscle injuries.

Improve Energy Levels

When you're exhausted the muscles become tighter and you will feel as if you'd like to lie down. If you get up and perform some stretches throughout your daytime routine You will discover that is an easy method to feel rejuvenated and feel more motivated to get more accomplished.

Improving Blood Flow

Stretching can naturally increase the flow of blood into the muscles that are sore. This can reduce your recovery time , and also prepare you for your next exercise.

Reduced Soreness

If you're only beginning an exercise routine, most likely you'll be a little more sore than an individual who has already been through itfor some time. However every athlete who is building their strength feel sore. The pain and swelling caused by muscles breaking and rebuilding to become stronger.

# Chapter 2: Weight Training To Lose Belly Fat

There's a clear distinction between fat loss and weight loss. Both are not identical. It is possible to lose weight or burning calories but there is no assurance that the weight that you've lost comes from the fat content.

Training for weights helps you shed the fat in specific parts of your body. Take your stomach, for instance since you can target specific areas of your body.

From the beginning losing weight may seem like an easy job. It is necessary to reduce the amount of calories you consume. However, the reality is more complex than that. To ensure that the weight you're losing is actually fat, you must have some regulation of hormones.

You must have a basic understanding of the physiology behind fat to comprehend this better.

There are receptors for every fat cell within your body. They're similar to tiny keyholes. They must be turned on in order to make your cell machinery shed fat. Hormones are what will open these receptors. They are catecholamine hormones that are responsible to eliminate belly fat. The body's system will experience a variety of physiological changes once the hormone is docked with its receptor in a fat cell. This is when you reduce the loss of muscle and reduce fat.

It is possible to burn lots of fat, however it's important to trigger catacholamine release to assist in burning fat effectively. The best way to achieve this is intense weight training.

Human Growth Hormone (HGH) and Lactic Acid

Catecholamine release and heavy weight training can be a pair. However, the catecholamine's action on the b-receptors are only the beginning.

Once catecholamine is released the body also produces blood sugar. In addition, when you burn sugar with high intensity exercise, oxygen supply is reduced. This produces an end-product, lactic acid. When the concentration of lactic acid rises it triggers the release of Human Growth Hormone or the HGH and testosterone hormone. It is now HGH as well as testosterone constitute two extremely powerful hormones that burn fat.

Testosterone increases the number of B-receptors to belly fat. HGH is the opposite. It stops cortisol from storage of fat. Together the two hormones help you lose more fat. Actually, once you have this process in place you'll keep losing belly fat in subsequent exercise sessions, too.

Study Reveals Amazing Results

Researchers at the East Carolina University carried out an investigation in the last few days. The results have been published in Journal of Applied Physiology.

The research revealed that weight training is capable of burning belly fat even after you've stopped working out. Probes were inserted into the subcutaneous belly fat within the participants. The probes were left there before , during, and after it, and for up to 15 min after weight-training. The subjects all completed the entire body resistance exercise which included three set of lifting weights, and 10 repetitions.

Researchers found that participants were more likely to use abdominal fat in their weight trainingand continued to use this for 40 minutes after exercising.

But it's not the only thing...

Another study has shown that it is possible to prevent the accumulation of fat due to age around the abdomen through weight training just twice a week. The study's findings is presented at the American Heart Association.

The researchers tracked over 164 overweight women for two years. They were split between two classes. One group was instructed to exercise every day for 30 minutes up to an hour, whereas the second group engaged in structured training for weights twice per week. The second group had more impressive results.

# Chapter 3: Callisthenic Workouts And Physiological Response Of The Body

The body's structure is designed to maintain equilibrium when you encounter a stressful circumstance or when you are subjected to a constant workout. The result is an aerobic and a higher cardiovascular endurance in every part of your body.

The Respiratory and Cardiovascular System

The principal functions for these systems within the body is to provide an uninterrupted flow of oxygen to all areas of the body, while simultaneously ridding the body of harmful carbon dioxide and transferring the necessary hormones to the proper sites and also regulating the supply of biochemical substances that are essential to the body.

The cardiovascular system of your body is composed by your heart. The heart is split in four compartments (the ventricles and the auricles) as well as the veins and arteries, as well as other vessels. The heart is subject to significant changes throughout the exercise that result in an improvement in flow to oxygen and nutrients and other essential elements to muscles and the areas of the body that require it. Alongside the supply of these elements, blood flow is concentrated in those parts of the body that are most active, such as the musculoskeletal system as well as the skin's surface. Since your heart's rate of activity and functions of the heart increase as a result of an increased need for oxygen and lung capacity gets increased as greater quantities of air are absorbed to allow it to satisfy the increasing demand for oxygen for the body at this point in time.

The Musculoskeletal System

It's the support system of the body, to which muscles are connected and also acts as a safeguard mechanism for the delicate organs and organs within the body. The muscles and skeleton responds to changing workout routines by increasing its capacity in storing energy. It's it is also more efficient in the utilization of oxygen to degrade these energies. Engaging in calisthenics exercises is an excellent way of building up your strength, increasing your reserves of energy and the intake of oxygen.

Common Terms employed in Workout Sessions

Calisthenics is a great way to make use of your bodyweight as there's no equipment involved. This method of exercise using your body weight demands cardio exercise and a core training strength, endurance, and a exercise, etc.

Active Rest are the breaks are taken in between or during your exercise session. It generally involves exercises that are moderate intensity contrasted to the training that you've just completed or set to undertake. Some examples of rest that are active include running continuously or stretching at a single spot.

Aerobic Exercises. The main goal on these workouts is build the cardiovascular and respiratory function of your lungs and your heart. This is achieved by the continuous motions of every body part, with slight variations in the speed at which you move.

It is a Bodyweight workout and Training This involves the use of various joints simultaneously e.g. presses up and pushups, squats, pushups, lunges, squats. The weight of your body is utilized to increase the endurance of muscles and increase its overall mass.

Cheat reps occur when you use an incorrect body park to perform training; this implies that you're cutting corners in order to meet your desired goals This will usually cause the entire workout to not being successful. It can also have serious consequences since there could be injuries as a result of an incorrect structure of the exercise that was not adhered to.

Circuits are the term that is used the moment you begin and finish an exercise session designed to increase your endurance and strength. The circuit is planned so that you need to check out the scheduled schedule of exercisesthat incorporates several different exercises before you move on to the next circuit.

Compound Movement, often referred to as the compound lift. It is an exercise that involves many muscles types from different areas of the body simultaneously. Consider the squat exercise routine for instance; it targets the muscles in the lower back, the back of the legs gluteus maximus. If you think about the pushup it targets the muscles in the upper portion of the body, such as shoulders, chests and the triceps.

Core Stability Workout exercise will help to build strength and improve your body's steady in movements, with the main concentration on the muscles in the mid-region (stomach and back, pelvis).

Form is the techniques used to engage and finishing the workout. The best form is one where you focus on specific muscles for the greatest actions and result from the exercise routine. Just like any workout it is essential to do it correctly to ensure that the targeted muscles are engaged fully and there aren't any injuries due to incorrect forms.

Missed Workout: This phrase refers to an event that a person fails to follow or is unable to follow a schedule of exercise. The most effective way to make sure that you are in sync with your fitness routines is to ensure that if an exercise session is skipped multiple times, your training should be re-run to reap the maximum benefit and not deceive yourself by skipping workouts or trying to skip certain elements of the workout.

Set and Repetitions. This is the total amount of times that the workout was performed. Repetition refers to a exercise movement e.g. for instance, when you're doing crunches 20 times. Sets are the amount of times you perform the repetition of a specific exercise e.g. for example, doing an entire set consisting of twenty crunches.

Tempo is the method or method you've decided to perform the exercise. It's the pace at which the various elements of your exercise are performed or the method you use to change between different areas of your body throughout the exercise. The ideal tempo is expressed in a ratio between 3:2 and 1 e.g. in the case of the crunch exercise is to go down into the crunch position, and staying in that position for 3 seconds. remain in that position for another 2 seconds , then returning back to the starting position for one second.

With these fundamental terms you're beginning to understand how to perform your calisthenics and exercises using your body weight.

# Chapter 4: Upper Body Exercises

The first and most important thing is to thank you for buying this book. I hope that you enjoy studying it. More important, you decide to pick the time to follow this easy exercise routine.

In the first chapter of this book we'll examine 20 upper body exercises that will assist you in getting fit shoulders and a toned chest. strengthen your muscles of your back.

Jumping Jacks

Jumping jacks is one of the most popular exercises across the world as they assist in warming the body, and provide the perfect cardio vascular exercise starting. The most popular type of jumping jack is their versatility and everyone of any age can do the exercise.

How to perform jumping jacks, must sit with your legs firmly joined and your arms at your sides. Then, you jump up and lift your hands over your head, then join them while your feet spread out and you land in an open position. After that, jump again and lower your arms towards your sides and connect your legs. Repeat this process.

What is the number of reps? You can begin your routine with jumping jacks . You can perform 200-300 reps based on your comfort level. Some prefer doing 150 reps at the start of their workout, and then 150 at the end for added leverage to their exercise.

Pros: This exercise aids in burning calories so that you'll lose weight easily. It also aids in increasing metabolic rate. It helps strengthen muscles in your abdominal and calves, and helps tone these regions. The jumping jacks can also help improve bones and enable you to keep a healthy body weight.

Planks

Planks are fantastic exercises for the upper body and are also considered to be total body exercises. They are an element of core workouts and will strengthen your abdominal muscles as well as build those muscles in your lower back. However, it is important to practice it in the right method to reap the full benefits.

To do planks, begin by standing up in an upright position , with your arms at your sides. Then, bend forward and then use fingers to lower the body of yours until it reaches the upper part of a push-up. Your toes should be supporting your legs, and your butt should point upwards. You can help the upper part of your body with your hands on the ground but some prefer to do it with their lower arms as it helps them keep the posture for longer. The body must be pulled back and then return to the standing position to finish the exercise. Repeat the sequence for those planks.

How many repetitions The recommended number of reps is 30 to 40 planks , depending on your comfort level and then hold each one at a 30-second interval.

Pros: This workout will benefit abdominal muscles. It will aid in sculpting your back and chest muscles. Your spine will experience a total stretch while your whole body is going to feel refreshed. Many people do this exercise to ease chronic back discomfort.

Mountain climbers

Mountain climbers are the next most effective upper body workout to do since it will aid in maximizing the benefits you get from your plank workouts. However, you don't have to do this sequence and you can choose to do mountain climbers prior to your planks.

How to do the mountain climber exercise first stand straight, with your hands at your side. After that take your body lower to reach the upper push up position, exactly as you would for the plank. Then, look straight ahead and lift your right leg towards your chest before pushing them back. Move your left knee upwards in the same manner, and then push it back. Then repeat the alternate leg movement until it feels like you're climbing the mountain.

How many repetitions: You can perform 20 repetitions of mountain climbers, and two to four sets, according to your comfort level.

Pros: Mountain climbers assist in strengthening abdominal muscles, as well as your chest. However, your back is the one that will reap the most benefit since from your back's upper to lower, this exercise can aid in strengthening and toning all the muscles. This exercise is great for your lungs and heart and, depending on the strength of your body you will be able to increase the intensity with each exercise.

Crunches

If someone wants to build up their stomachs and build up their upper body muscles the first exercise that comes to thoughts is crunches. Crunches are among the best exercises you can do for strength in the upper body since they assist in sculpting the chest and shoulder muscles. They can also be beneficial for neck muscles and reduce neck pain.

What to do The following are the different types of crunches however we will concentrate on two major varieties viz. the classic crunch along with the cycle crunch.

The crunch that is the foundation

The fundamental crunch can be performed by first lying down on the ground with your legs together and your arms to your sides. Then, put your hands on your neck. You may also raise the neck to the ceiling. Fold your legs over and keep a small distance between your butt and heel. Then slowly lift your upper body until you are able to attempt to touch your knees using your elbows. If you're lifting your hands, you can stretch them in front over your knees. Return to the starting position after holding the posture for a few minutes. Repeat the fundamental crunch.

The crunch of the bicycle

For the bicycle crunch you'll need to lay down the same way like you would for the standard crunch. After that, you should put your legs on the floor and put your hands under your head. For the crunch, pull your knees to your chest, and then lift your upper body in a single motion. You can now you will twist your back to left, and then raise your left leg. As you twist, reach your left knee with the right hand. Repeat the opposite side.

What is the number of reps Do you need to do? You can complete 15 reps, and 4 sets for an overall total of 60. You can perform 30 standard as well as 30 bike crunches.

Pros: Crunches work for your entire body, but they are especially beneficial for the abdominals, chest and shoulders. The neck and shoulder muscles will be able to fully flex and any discomfort will ease.

Hot feet

Hot feet are an exercise in cardio that aids the upper body to get an entire workout. This is usually done for the final part of the routine.

How to do hot feet, sit with your legs together with your hands close to your side. Then, you should spread your legs apart and bent a bit. Make sure your palms are tightly clenched and begin to move your legs upwards and downwards as quick as you are able to. In other words, you need to be able to bend your knees a bit and begin to run as fast as you can. Then, try to raise your knees to the highest level you can.

How many repetitions: It is possible to do this for anywhere from 3 to 5 minutes , and then try to have a 1-minute break between.

Pros: This workout is great for finishing your upper body workout because it helps your entire body move and help the muscles to relax. It lets your chest, shoulders and upper stomach to experience shaking, which will aid in burning off calories.

# Chapter 5: Exercises To Perform Using Common Household Items

Although many enjoy and find it enjoyable to exercise in an exercise facility but there are a few who prefer to sweat an intense workout in their home. In the end, all you require to get moving is you body, amount of determination, and a small pieces of household equipment. You'll be amazed by the ways you can make use of the most basic items you will find around your home.

1. Push-ups? No Problem! Use the Stairs!

It's probably one of the most used areas of the home. Push-ups are a great way to strengthen your upper body and the core muscles. Doing it on the stairs adds variety and variety to the push-up workout.

How do I do it?

Do a pushup however, this time are facing the stairs with your feet touch the floor.

Your hands should be placed just below the shoulders and your abs must be tight. Bring your body down to about an inch from the stairs, then keep your pulse low for two to three times, and then push yourself up.

2. Squatting with one leg with the chair

Another common item used at home includes the chair. Did you know that it could also be an ideal exercise device?

What can you do?

Sitting Position

Put a chair that is about one foot in front of you and then stand. Make sure to support yourself with the help from your leg. Slowly raise the right leg as well as both arms in the direction of your body. Then bend your left knee , and lower yourself until you're sitting down on the chair. Then, stop for a moment and before driving back to your beginning position.

Standing Position

You could also stand in the seat and sit on your left leg , keeping one foot on of the chair with you arms out straight. Turn your left knee to the side and then sit back into the squat for as long as you are able. Return to your the starting position. This can be a little challenging and requires stability.

1. Do you not have dumbbells? Two bottles of water will suffice!

Doing your workout at home can be an even better option since you don't have waiting for gym equipment to be accessible as you would in an exercise facility. You could even use bottles of water to replace dumbbells. Make sure to fill them up with water.

How do I do it?

Start in a position where you will be standing on your feet, and your hands hold 1.5 Liters of water from a bottle. When you raise the bottles up, you should contract your abdominal muscles. Lower the hands that are behind you, placing your elbows close the ear. The bottles should be lifted up, while you move your left leg towards the side. Start to release and then do 3 reps for each leg.

2. Don't let the stability ball rest in your storage room.

Utilizing an stability ball during your routine of home exercise is another way to strengthen your back and mid-section. It will allow your core to get tighter and open up for the movements that are appropriate to be used in certain exercises. By using a stabilization ball you can do ab curly as well as hamstring curls, bench presses and presses.

What can you do?

Shins should be set onto the balance ball. Keep your hands are on the floor until you are in a planking posture. When you're in the planking position you can walk your hands as your shins are in the air. Keep your abs strong. To make the workout more difficult, walk using your hands and gradually raise your leg to the side. Release the leg and repeat the same process by using you right leg.

3. On the bed

Who says that the bed is just for rest? It could be a workout place too.

4. What can you do?

This simple exercise focuses on those muscles in the middle. It is regarded as a fundamental move since it requires the muscles to be more intense in order to be solid on the soft bed. Start by lying on your back with legs and arms lifted towards the ceiling. Then reduce your legs and arms simultaneously until they are just a few inches away from the mattress. Repeat the steps and make sure you keep the core in place.

# Chapter 6: Types Of Exercises And Fitness Terms You Have To Know

As I've mentioned in my previous article, many people who would like to start exercising do not realize what they're doing. It is crucial to get all the information you can about working out in the best way you are able to. It is an excellent idea to educate yourself. idea. Learn everything you can and reap the benefits from it in the long run.

Types of Exercises

A well-balanced fitness regimen includes various kinds of exercises based on the goals you have set. If, for instance, you are looking to shed weight, your program should include a combination of cardio and strength training in order to help you lose weight. Professional athletes stay away from accidents by focussing on strengthening.

If you're looking to establish an exercise routine that is suitable for your needs and goals, you must be familiar with these various types of workouts.

Cardio/Aerobic Exercise

Based on the two Greek words Aero-air and Bios which translates to living, aerobic exercise is the kind of exercise that increase the body's need to get oxygen. Aerobic exercises like running, walking fast cycling, swimming and aero dancing are intense enough to require your body to increase the heart rate and breathing. Also known as cardiovascular This type of exercise can helps keep your heart and lungs in good shape and contributes to overall wellness of your body.

Strength Training

If you are looking to build your muscles and increase your body's resistance, this is the kind of exercise you need to incorporate into your workout routine. The exercises that fall in this category include the lifting of weights using bands of resistance or any other physical activity that's against your body weight, such as walking up stairs or doing push-ups. Strength training can help reduce the fat in your body to be more leaner and stronger muscles. Other benefits that this workout can bring include building strong bones, increasing strength, and weight control.

Flexibility Exercises

While strengthening exercises are focused on muscles, stretching exercises focus on giving joints a wider mobility. By doing these exercises, including stretching, yoga, or stretching your calf muscles will help you gain more flexibility, which might be diminished due to age. If you're having difficulty getting things off the floor or getting to the top of your cabinet Then flexibility training could aid you tremendously.

Balance Exercising

Balance is among the essential factors is required to exercise particularly if your body is limiting you in your daily tasks. Being able to maintain a good hand-eye coordination and balance will allow you to maintain the body's functions. This is why this kind of exercise is crucial to combat the effects of aging. A few of the exercises that fall into this category are one-leg balance and heel-to-toe exercise.

Fitness Terms to Know

You're already familiar with the various types of exercise, but it's essential to be familiar with the various fitness terms.

Warm-up

This is a practice you follow prior to beginning the actual exercise. The importance of warm-ups is that they prepare your body, your muscles and tendons to handle the intense physical activities that lie ahead. They help you avoid injuries and maximizes the benefits of working out. Stretching, toe touch as well as knee and hip circles are typically part of the warm-up routine.

Cool down

The cooling down routine is as crucial as the warm-up routine. Because your heart rate higher during intense workouts cooling down can help in bringing your body back to its normal state of relaxation. By stretching the muscles that you exercised keeps them in a good shape and reduce the chance of injury.

Heart Rate

The monitoring of your heartbeat during exercise is crucial to ensure your safety. Since your heart rate can increase (from 30 beats/minute to between 60 and 100 beats/minute) during exercise it's crucial to know whether the workout is suitable for you. If you surpass your heart rate's maximum when you exercise it is obvious that you must take the intensity down. (A max heart rate can be calculated by subtracting your years of age by 220. E.g. 220-45yrs. old= 175 maximum heart rate)

Repetitions (Reps)

This refers to the amount of repetitions you do an exercise within the course of a set. For instance, if you do 50 sit-ups. Then you performed 50 reps on the sit-up workout.

Set

A set, however, is the number of times you complete the exercise. For instance, you might do 10 repetitions of lifting weights before taking a break to prepare for a new "set" of lifting weights.

If you're looking to get serious about exercising, I suggest to familiarize yourself with the terms of fitness however these are the essentials you need to begin.

# Chapter 7: Lower Body Exercises Without Equipment

The lower part of your body needs exactly the same amount of work as your upper body , and in some cases, even more.

The six-pack abs only be achieved when you do the right type of lower-body exercises and here are some of the most effective that you can do without equipment.

Supine pose/ Spinal twist

The supine posture is a stretch for your lower body posture that assists by stretching the spine as well as the muscles of your lower back, and prepare you for the next exercises. The exercise appears simple, but it will give your body a full workout, and will stretch your muscles to ease any tension in your back or butt. The twist in your spine will make you feel refreshed and ready for the rest of your routine.

How to do the supine posture to sleep, lie in a position on your floor, with feet together and your hands at your sides. Lift your legs up to 90 degrees and then join your heels in the air. As much as you can, and then gradually lower them until that your knees are bent. Then slowly push them up and repeat.

For the spine twist, stretch your legs out to the side on the flooring. Then, you can roll your right leg on your left, and then bend it. Make use of your right hand press it down while your right hand will extend outward. It will feel like a total stretch of the spine. Repeat the opposite side.

How many repetitions You can do these for 5 minutes, without break.

Pros: This posture is a fantastic option to start your lower body workouts. It will allow your muscles to relax and put you more comfortable for stretching your muscles.

Squat swing Jack

Like the name implies, this workout will require you to do three actions at a time. It's designed in order to offer your legs an entire exercise and to also let your upper body gain some benefits.

How to complete this exercise, sit with your legs together with your hands close to your side. Then, jump as you would in a jumping jack, however you make your landing much more wide and then squat. Put your right hand between your legs. place your feet on the floor using your fingers. Then, push your right hand back as far as you can in order to twist your body. Do this for a few seconds before jumping with your legs together and lifting your right arm upwards. Repeat the same exercise with your second hand, making sure you alternate hands as you repeat the repetitions.

The number of reps you can do: 15 reps, and 4 to five sets based on your level of comfort.

Pros: This workout is excellent because it will strengthen your abs, strengthen your thighs, and trigger your butt muscles to get firmer. Your shoulders and hands will feel the heat and your back muscles will be able to flex.

Pike push up

The pike press up is a variation on the push up that is generally used designed to give your upper and lower body with a full workout. This is a great exercise to complement your lower-body routine since it will increase the stretch of your lower back, and butt muscles.

What to do: Begin by standing straight, with your arms close to your sides. Then, lower to the plank and keep the upper push-up position. Slowly walk your hands back , and then jet your butt up. It is important to bend your back enough so that your spine can be straight. Then bend your elbows in such a way that your head drops and then bend until your head is almost touching the ground , then back up.

What reps are you able to do Do you need to do? 15 reps, and 5 sets.

Pros: This posture is perfect for your lower abdominals as you will feel the warmth. It is also possible to place the feet on a taller platform to help your abdominals to tone up.

Cobra pose

The cobra pose was created to aid your lower back muscles to get an entire stretch. It will aid in bringing your abs up.

How to practice this pose it is necessary to lie on the ground , with your hands at your sides and your belly pressed to the floor. Then, lift your head up and then use the hands of your arms to pull your upper body upwards. Keep your eyes upwards and allow your lower body to remain fixed to the floor. You should feel the abdominal muscles of your lower abdomen tingle and fully stretch.

What is the number of reps? Do 10 repetitions of this posture 5 times, and hold the upper position for five seconds per time.

Pros: This pose aids in stretching out your muscles in your chest, shoulders and the lower abdominal region. It aids in strengthening your muscles around your butt and is a great position for women because it eases menstrual cramps.

The warrior pose

This pose, called the warrior one is one that is borrowed that is from the yoga world. This pose can be a fantastic option to end your lower body exercises since it helps your body absorb the benefits that come from the rest of the postures.

How to do the warrior pose you should be standing with your legs joined and your arms at your sides. Slowly move your right leg forward to create lunge. Then, pull your left leg inwards. Take both hands up and place them together to your head on top. It is possible to look up at your hands that are joined and hold the position for a few seconds. Try to get as low as you can in order to allow your lower body to stretch to the maximum.

Another posture you could try is to stand straight and connect your hands over your head. Then, bend your knees and look down at the floor. Then slowly lift your right leg so that it is directly parallel to the floor. Keep it there for a few minutes before returning to your original position. repeat the exercise with the other leg.

How many repetitions Do you need to do? You can perform these warrior poses repeatedly as often as you'd like, and the number of reps will be based on the level of your comfort.

Pros: These postures are designed to give your lower body strength and increase the strength of your core muscles, as well as your butt and things.

# Chapter 8: How Muscle Growth Works

If you've found the gym, now it's time to master how to use those equipments to trigger some significant growth. What can you do to get your muscles to expand? How do you accomplish this in inside the convenience of your home , without the support or advice you'd get from training in a professional gym? Let's at...

The Basics

In order to build up muscle it is essential to stimulate hypertrophy. This is the technical term used for growing muscle and it usually happens when you're in a state of rest. It's the process of building muscle in two parts. The first part is the workout that breaks down muscle and allows it to be marked for growth . Part two is the growing stage which takes place after you've lifted while you're at rest.

This could happen by two different ways. This is:

Myofibrillar Hypertrophy

And

Sarcoplasmic Hypertrophy

The exact basis of these theories remains being debated and some claim that they are not accurate descriptions. But anyone who is a bodybuilder will explain that generally there are two methods to build muscle which appear to coincide with these ideas.

Two ways to do this are:

Muscle Damage

And

Metabolic Stress

In addition, there is another aspect at play, and that is the capacity to build strength. Strength is not always linked to the size of your muscles. Another aspect that is in the equation and which you have to consider is:

Muscle Fiber Recruitment

Okay. That's a lot of terms I've just thrown at you. What does each one mean?

Simply stated your muscles comprise a lot of tiny strands known as muscle fibers. They are actually cells exactly like the cells that comprise the other parts of your body as well as the neurons that compose your brain. This means they contain nuclei, which indicates that they are Sarcoplasma (if you have a good memory of the biology class you took in high school). ...).

The distinction is that muscles have numerous nuclei. They also have the capability to telescope to expand and contract. When this happens in mass the muscles to expand and contract as well and that is why you can lift objects at the gym.

There isn't a method to increase the number of muscle fibers. This is known as "hyperplasia and is only recognized to occur in very uncommon situations. What one can accomplish is disintegrate the muscle to allow it to grow more robust. It is accomplished by lifting heavy weights until exhaustion and, in particular, under tension and at that point, you cause microtears in the muscles. Proteins then help repair the tears. This is why the muscles to grow larger. This is also the reason for "DOMS," which is a delayed onset soreness in the muscles. This is why you could have difficulty lifting one cup of coffee the next morning...

This is known as myofibrillar hypertrophy, which is a result of the damage to muscles. The primary factor is to overwork the muscles. There are other elements to consider however, such as making sure you exercise muscles from a variety of angles in order to target every fiber, and training in both slow and fast forms to develop the slow and fast fibers.

Fast twitch fibers kick into action when slow twitch fibers don't have the capacity of lifting. These are by nature the strongest and strongest fibers that are found in your muscles. This is why you must have at minimum a certain amount of weight in order to stimulate these fibers.

So , what exactly does sarcoplasmic Hypertrophy include? It's a type of the growth of muscles due to swelling of the muscles by introducing fluids. If you exercise for a long period of time then you slowly pump your muscle with blood. This will rev the lactic acid system which fill them with chemicals as well. That is that the area of your body operating will get swollen from oxygen, blood, nutrients and energy. If you continue lifting, that triggers the muscle to get bigger and fuller , which then blocks the region (like applying a tourniquet to it).

The best part is that this causes an increase in metabolites which are compounds that promote growth like growth hormone or testosterone. Additionally muscles are more efficient in storage of glycogen and sarcoplasm in order to be able to perform for long periods. This results in a more 'puffy and 'looking' muscle that can last longer instead of a more brittle and more compact muscle that could produce more power in the short term.

It is also known as sarcoplasmic Hypertrophy and it is caused through metabolic stress. The main factor in bringing this about is the amount of time in tension, and it can cause the feeling of pumping in the fitness center.

Both kinds of training are effective and when you mix both types of training you can increase your size and strength. In general the bodybuilders exercise more using sarcoplasmic approaches while powerlifters employ more myofibrillar techniques.

And then there are those who affirm that there isn't anything called sarcoplasmic Hypertrophy. It does not matter. Consider this as a helpful mental tool to understand the process. In all times, fitness enthusiasts realize that lifting weights in small reps is a sign of greater power, whereas lifting lighter for higher reps is a sign of strength. Combining both is known as 'powerbuilding'.

There is one more thing we need to be aware of that is the recruitment of muscle fibers. Since if you study people like Bruce Lee, you'll see that it's possible to be extremely powerful without needing to possess an enormous amount of muscle mass. How? Through using a higher proportion of your muscle fibers in every move. Bruce Lee was the master of this, but there are numerous ways to train to increase control over the muscles.

The most important thing is to work at the top end of what you're able to do in terms of resistance. This causes your body to use all of your most powerful fibers of twitch in your muscle as is possible, which in turn strengthens the 'neuromuscular junction' in order to boost your power output. Bruce Lee would even use the technique known as static contraction. He would pull or push at an impervious force in order to train his body to generate as much force as he could.

Incorporate this in your everyday routine, and you'll be even more dangerous.

# Chapter 9: Single Leg Raise Pushup

Step 1

Start in an incline position (quadruped) in the yoga mat, placing your hands placed directly beneath your shoulders, your fingers facing forward and knees below your hips. Engage your abdominals and pull your shoulders downwards.

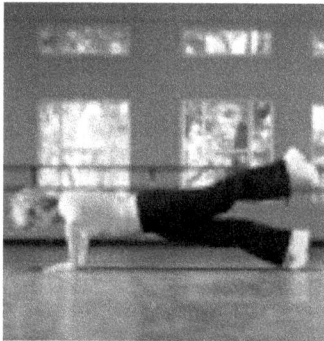

Step 2

Take one leg and then away, followed by the second leg, getting you into a the plank position. Engage your abdominals and core to support the body. Head should remain in alignment in line with the spine. Your feet should be positioned together with your toes snugly under , and your heels pointing towards the wall in front of you.

## Step 3

The Downward phase: slowly bend your elbows, then lower your body towards the floor. Maintain your torso in a straight line and your head in line to your spine. Don't allow your lower back or ribcage area to drop or your hips rise up. Utilize the glutes (butt) and quadriceps (thigh) muscles to maintain stability and a strong body. Make sure at lowering yourself till your chin or chest reach the floor or mat. Your elbows should be in close proximity to each other, or allow them to extend outwards slightly.

## Step 4

Upward Phase: Straighten your elbows by pressing upwards with your arms. Maintain your torso straight and your the head in alignment to your spine. As you straighten your arms then lift your left foot off the floor, while keeping your knee straight. Make sure that your hips are not allowed to turn as you lift your leg from the ground. Don't let your low back or ribcage to slide as your hips rise up. Keep pressing until your elbows remain straight, and the left foot is lifted off the floor. You should hold this position for a short time before returning to the starting position. Repeat the push-up, alternating legs after each repetition.

The heel and the outside of your palm will increase the force of your press , and also the stability of your shoulders.

Front Plank

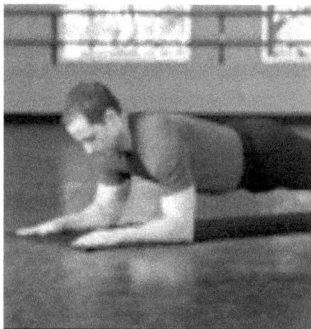

Step 1

Starting Position: Lay in a stomach position on flooring or an exercise mat with your elbows near your sides, and directly beneath your shoulders with your palms downwards and your fingers in front. Involve your abdominal/core muscles. It should feel as if you're tying an elastic band around your waist, ribs, as well as your lower back. Engage your thigh muscles in order to stretch your legs firmly and then flex your ankles (tucking your toes toward the shins).

Step 2

Upward Phase. Slowly lift your thighs and your torso off the mat or floor. Maintain your legs and torso in a straight position. Avoid sliding in your ribcage, or lower back. Do not lift your hips up to the sky or bending your knees. Keep your shoulders clear of your ears (no shrugging). Your shoulders should be straight over your elbows , with your palms down throughout the entire workout. Maintain your breathing and keep your abdominal muscles strong while in this position. Try to hold this position for five to ten seconds or more.

Step 3

Downwards Phase: Keep the legs and torso straight in order to slowly lower the body towards the mat or the floor.

Side Plank with Bent Knee

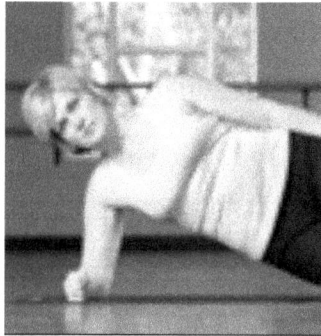

Step 1

Start Position: Lay on your back lying on a mat, knees bent. You can also have your legs stacked one over each other in a comfortable posture. Work your core and abdominal muscles while you raise your torso and then rest your body by the right side of your forearm. Right elbow should be bent. It should rest directly beneath your shoulder. The head must be in alignment in line with the spine. Your lower leg and hips are on the exercise mat.

Step 2

Inhale and exhale upwards and keep the abdominal muscles tight to stabilize the spine. Head should remain in alignment with your spine.

Step 3

Lowering Phase: Inhale , and slowly return to your original position. After a predetermined number of times, repeat the opposite side.

Step 4

Variations to Exercise: You may increase the intensity of your workout by increasing the duration of time that you're in the elevated position.

Supine Reverse Crunches

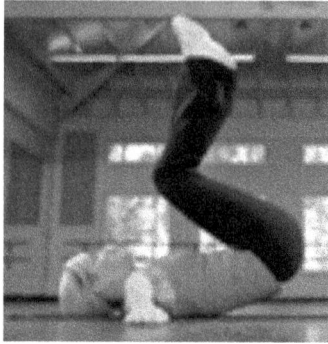

## Step 1

Start in a comfortable position: lie on your mat on your back and bend your knees. feet laid flat on the ground and arms spread toward your sides, your palms facing downwards. Relax gently. Involve your abdominal and core muscles to support your spine. Then slowly raise your heels off of the floor, and then raise your knees straight over your hips. The knees should be bent 90 degrees. Maintain this position while breathing normally. Utilize your arms as a source of support.

## Step 2

Upward Phase: Inhale and slowly lift your hips off of the mat. Roll your spine upwards as if you were trying to draw your knees toward your head. Make sure to not alter the knee's angle when you roll them up. Utilize your arms and hands to assist in maintaining your balance. Continue to roll up until your spine can't continue to roll. Do this for a short time.

Step 3

The Downward phase: Gently inhale. As you control your breathing, lower your hips and spine back to your starting position.

A proper form is crucial in this exercise in order to avoid putting too much strain on your lower back. As you return to your starting position you must control the movement of your legs. Don't let your knees slide beyond your hips, but instead, return to a position that is directly over your hips. Since abdominal muscles connect your rib cage to your pelvis, you should make sure that the primary focus of your exercise should be to pull your pelvis upwards toward your rib cage.

Cobra

Step 1

Start Position: Lay with your back on flooring or an exercise mat with your hands just below your shoulders, with your fingers in front. Your legs should be straight with your toes directed.

Step 2

The Upward phase: Gently exhale. Engage your abdominal muscles and core muscles to assist the spine. Place your hips on the mat or the floor. Then, lengthen your torso and pull your shoulders away from the ground as you keep your hips steady. Keep your shoulders moving down and back. Maintain this position for 15 to 30 minutes.

Step 3

Downward Phase Begin by gently lowering your upper body back down to the floor or mat while lengthening your spine as you descend.

Squat Jumps

Step 1

Start in a standing position with your feet about hip-width apart, your arms at your sides. Bring your shoulder blades downwards and contract your abdominal or core muscles to stabilize your spine.

Step 2

Downward phase: Slide your hips forward and downwards. This will result in the appearance of a hinge between your knees. Keep lowering yourself until your heels feel ready to lift off of the floor. Be sure to maintain a straight rear by leaning forward at your hips. Keep your head facing towards the front and place your arms so that they provide the highest amount of balance support.

Step 3

Jumping Movement: After one very short gap at the bottom of your downwards phase and then explode upwards through your lower body, completely extending your knees, hips and ankles. While you leap to the sky, you should try keeping your heels aligned with one another and parallel to the floor.

Step 4

Landing: The primary aspects of landing are a correct foot placement and avoiding overly forward movement within your lower extremity which puts additional strain to your knees.

Step 5

Make sure to land gently and gently on the mid-foot before rolling to the heels. Always pull your hips back and lower to cushion the force of landing. Don't lock your knees when landing.

Step 6

Your trunk should be slightly forward, with your head in alignment with your spine and back flat or rigid. Keep your abdominal or core muscles active and bracing your torso to help protect your spine.

# Chapter 10: Full Body - Home

Workout Plan

RULES. This workout should be done for 6-8 weeks. Then , you can begin your SPLIT exercise. Whatever the goal you are trying to achieve - to lose weight, gain muscles and tone up your the body. The principles are the same. This full-body workout can be effective for those who want to build muscle or shed fat (when you're trying to lose fat, perform another one to three aerobic sessions and break for shorter intervals during sets).

Stay on the program for a long time and you'll be happy and those around will notice the changes. The initial effects are already evident after just three weeks. After 90 days, your body may change beyond the point of. The plan is displayed in textual and graphic format.

There Is No Shortcuts. Just Do The Work

How To Train With This System

Perform this exercise 3-4 times a week. Every other or third day.

Example;

* Monday; (workout)

* Tuesday; Rest Day

* Wednesday; (workout)

* Thursday; Rest Day

* Friday; (workout)

* Saturday; Rest Day

* Sunday; (workout)

And and so to...

Complete the exercises one at a time. If you're a beginner begin with fewer sets of each exercise, and less repetitions. The breaks between series should not last more than 30 seconds. If the weight you are working with is too light, add more weight to the weight. If you find the entire workout challenging, don't be concerned, just perform as many exercises as you are able to. Try to increase the number of exercises in your next exercise. Make sure you do at least 15 sets per workout.

Good Luck!

To achieve the best results, adhere to the previously established assumptions.

- Set a Goal,

- Calculate Caloric Needs,

- Train According to the Established Workout Plan,

- Stick to Diet Assumptions, and Count Calories

- Track the Effects

Track a Training Progress

This journal lets you monitor the effect of your training. Make sure to utilize this tool during each workout. It is possible to use the charts to monitor your progress in training by using two methods. The first is to conduct the training according to the schedule you've made for the coming weeks. After each exercise, you input it into the table, along with your number of reps you completed and the weight you worked on. Another way to make use of tables is to arrange the training session prior to your beginning your training. Simply, prior to each workout , enter the number of reps you'll be doing today and using the weight. In what reps and sets.

# Chapter 11: Weight Training Exercises To Lose Weight

Here are some fantastic exercises to strengthen your body that you need to do.

Barbell Squat

The Barbell squat works on the muscles in your legs. Maintain your feet on the ground with firmness. The feet must be at a shoulder width apart. Then, keep a barbell on the upper portion of your back. It should be placed comfortably. Avoid your neck. Keep the bar about 1 foot from your shoulders. Step away from the barbell rack. Lower your shoulders and strengthen your core. Begin to squat gradually until your quadriceps muscles are in line and in line with your ground. Press yourself to get back to a standing position. Repeat the exercise for a few seconds.

It is vital to keep a the correct posture during every squat. Maintain the back straight. You shouldn't bend your back, as it could result in an injury to your back.

Barbell Squat

Dumbbell Swing

The exercise target the muscle in your shoulders. Make sure you stand slightly higher than shoulder width. The dumbbell should be at your side and on your floor. Squat now. Make sure your core is tight and secure the dumbbell using your palm. It should face you. Maintain your back straight while you lift your legs up with power. Then, you can swing the dumbbell upwards in direction towards the ceiling until it's just above the eyes.

Maintain your posture. Lower the weight to the floor in a quick and fluid movement. Repeat the motion 12 times before switching to the opposite arm.

Dumbbell Swing

Dumbbell Front Squat

When you are starting the feet must be placed shoulder-width apart. Place a dumbbell between your hands. Then lower your body. Make sure the dumbbells are placed in front of your shoulders. Your palms should face one opposite. Your weight should be placed on your heels. Stop when your hamstrings are aligned with the ground. Your back and core must be in a straight line. Keep your chin straight to the ground. This exercise can strengthen your biceps and hamstrings as well as your bicep and quadriceps. It's easy and efficient.

Dumbbell Front Squat

Single-Leg Dumbbell Row

This workout is designed for your abs, hamstrings quadriceps, butt, shoulders, biceps, and back.

Place your feet on the floor with a five to 10 pounds mass in the left of your hand. Then, you can pivot forward, ensuring that your back is level and in line with the floor.

Find support by holding a low table or chair with your left hand. Then, extend your left arm toward the floor. Keep your palms in the direction of your left foot. Then, lift your left leg in front of your back. Your body should be in an "T" position.

Relax your left elbow slowly. Lift the weight until you're elbow's in an a level position with your the torso. Lower the weight once you have held it for a second. Perform 15 repetitions prior to switching sides.

Single-Leg Dumbbell Row

Kettlebell Swings

Kettlebells are balls from cast iron. They have a single handle inside these kettlebells. In contrast to traditional weights you must be able to hold of kettlebells isn't distributed equally. This means you must put in more effort to support your body in order that the weight of the kettlebell is balanced.

Utilize both hands to hold the kettlebell, keeping your feet at a shoulder width. Extend your arms to the max and do a squat. The weight should rest between your legs. Place the kettlebell to the side and under your feet. Push your hips forward as you lift the weight towards your chest. Your arms should be straight during this exercise. Lower the weight. You should be able to pass it under your. Perform a few repetitions. Keep in mind that you shouldn't do anything that causes you to arch or turn your back.

Kettlebell swings are extremely beneficial since this workout combines aerobic and anaerobic exercise to help burn calories. You'll definitely be able to shed weight.

This workout can be performed using a dumbbell, too.

Kettlebell Swings

Squat to Overhead Press

This workout is designed to strengthen your shoulders, abs butt, hamstrings and quadriceps.

Maintain the feet of your hands shoulder width apart while you stand. The elbows must be bent. You should hold a weight of 5 pounds in both hands. Make sure that the weight is at the shoulder's height. Your palms should point toward the front. Then lower yourself to an squatting position. Be sure to ensure that your knees don't go over your toes. Keep this posture and count to three.

You can push your heels to the point of getting up while you lift the weights above you. Return to your starting position. Do it 15 more times.

*Squat to Overhead Press*

*Dolphin Plank*

This workout strengthens your shoulders, abs, and the back muscles.

Lay down on the floor with your head down. Keep your toes tucked. Bring the bellybutton into your spine, even though your forearms are lying on the floor. Your hips should be raised until they are in the lowest plank position.

Breathe in as you are raising your legs. Your body should take on an reversed "V" position. Take a break for a second. Return to the beginning position. Perform three sets of 15 each.

Dolphin Plank

Lower Abs Trifecta

This workout targets the muscles in your lower abdominals. It's an excellent exercise to lose belly fat and keeping it off in the long term. It's actually a combination of three lower abdominal exercises such as Reverse Crunches Ab V Holds, as well as Abs Pulse Ups.

First do the Abs Pulse Ups. Place your body on your back and sit on the bench for weight lifting or on the floor. Place your hands under your hips when you are doing this in a floor. But if you're doing this on a table the hands must be in the same position as your head. Lift your legs while you strengthen your core. You should have your legs at 90 degrees with your body. Now , squeeze your butt while lowering your the abs. Bring your legs towards your hips. Don't bend your legs. Keep them for a moment and then slowly lower until you are near your butt. Repeat the set. 15 repetitions is enough.

Moving to Reverse Crunches the next. Keep your back straight and maintain your legs in the place on the table. Place your hands close to your head when you're at the bench. Work your lower abs to the max and keep your upper back in a neutral position. Lift your butts off the floor and bring the knees towards your head. Make sure to hold for a second after your knees are high to the chest. Return to the beginning position. It is also possible to put an exercise ball between your feet to make it harder.

The next one is Abs V Hold. Lay on your back and lie down. Lift your legs and raise your upper body simultaneously while contracting your abs muscles. Your body should create a "V" shape. The angle between your torso as well as your legs should be at least 45 degrees. Keep your legs straight. Your posture should be solid during this workout. Utilize your hands to hold your knees as long as you are able to. Return to your beginning position gradually.

Complete these three exercises , one after the next without resting.

Lower Abs Trifecta

Step up your game by incorporating Bicep Curl

This is where you're engaging the muscles of your biceps and butt, quadriceps, hamstrings, and abs.

Keep your left foot on a bench. Place 5 pounds of weight in both hands. Place pressure on your left foot while you attempt to raise yourself. Keep your right thigh elevated to make sure it's directly parallel to the floor. The weight should be lifted to your shoulders simultaneously. Return to your starting position. Switch sides after 15 repetitions. Three sets should suffice.

Step up with Bicep Curl

Curtsy Lunge

This workout targets the abs muscles as well as quadriceps, hamstrings butt and hips.

Keep your hands on your hips when you stand with your feet about hip width apart. Take a step back in a diagonal direction using one foot on the left. This is crossed behind your right. Flex your knees when you lower your left hand towards the floor. Make sure you reach the outside portion on your left foot using the left side of your hand.

Return to the position from which you started. Switch sides after 15 repetitions. Three repetitions of the exercise.

Curtsy Lunge

Cross Fit

Cross Fit is great for those who have lifted weights for some time. Sure, it will help you shed weight, but novices should avoid this to avoid it for the future. It involves a variety of routines of exercise like exercise for endurance weight lifting speed and strength training as well as plyometric and kettlebell exercises among other things. It is always interesting by this exercise, since Cross Fit is actually several exercises that are incorporated into one fat-burning exercise.

It targets all the important fitness-related components of physical fitness, such as endurance, speed, flexibility cardiovascular fitness, and power.

It is possible to do 30 push-upsand 20 pull-ups, 50 squats along with 40 sit-ups. It is possible to mix the exercises in order to keep it engaging. Repeat each one. Pause for 3 minutes between each repetition.

Cross Fit is extremely effective in burning calories and fat. It boosts endurance, boosts metabolism, and physical stamina as well.

The whole workout shouldn't last longer than 15 or 20 minutes.

Cross Fit

Turkish Getup

Lay on your back and lie down. Spread your right hand over the chest. Your right foot must remain completely level to the floor. Extend your left leg completely. Place your left hand in the ground. Apply pressure to the abdominal muscles while you sit up. Make use of your left and right feet to lift yourself off the ground. Move your left leg under your body when lifting to get yourself in your lunge posture. Get up and push through your heels as you are moving your feet together side by side. This exercise can benefit your legs, core and shoulders.

Turkish Getup

Circuit Routine

It is possible to tone your problematic areas and burn fat effectively by combining weight machines and free-weight exercises. When you train in circuits you must complete every exercise and have minimal rest between them. In this case, you're doing one exercise on one machine and after that, switching to the next without stopping for too long, yet they are both part of this same exercise. In the end, you will spend approximately 10 minutes on the cardio machine.

Leg extensions and leg curls and leg presses to strengthen the lower portion of your physique. Perform triceps dumbbell extension exercises for the back of your arms, as well as dumbbell curls to strengthen your Biceps. The dumbbell military press should strengthen your shoulders' muscles. Do side bends as well as double crunches to strengthen your waist. Perform 8-12 repetitions of each for at least four rounds. Increase your weight after just a few repetitions. As you continue, you'll lose more fat.

This exercise can be done two times per week.

# Chapter 12: Maximizing The Results Of The Workout

The primary goal of your calisthenics and bodybuilding exercises is to build the strength and development of your muscles. While doing this you could also utilize it to boost the strength and endurance of your body. The ability to maximize your workout time is the main goal that is what controls and determines the priority of each move. If the motivation and enthusiasm is not channeled properly to the right form of exercise, using the right technique and technique, you could be injured and possibly not see the improvement in muscle tone you've always hoped for. It's not enough to just lie on your couch, snacking all day long and watching television with the hope that you can get those abs that are ribbed and toned simultaneously. You must put in the effort and provide an amount of commitment to your exercise routine in order in order to get fit.

All done, how do you make the most of your workouts? The first thing you need to know is the type of workout you'd like to do as well as the correct way to do it as well as the wide range of food items that you must eat and lastly, the things are not recommended and that you must take on to achieve positive results.

Timing and Duration of Workouts

It is not possible to get up and go exercising without a plan for doing so. It is essential to have a clearly planned out schedule of the days and hours of the day you plan to work out and the kind of exercise to carry out on the scheduled dates, the duration and intensity, as well as kind of food that you will consume prior to and after your exercise. With a set time that you can easily manage it can aid to ensure that you adhere to the time and adhere to the program.

If you're a novice you are likely that you'll have lots of motivation and the time you have set for your workouts could be somewhat unrealistic and unrealistic. This could result in you not meeting your targets , leading to unsuccessful exercises, and motivation levels will plummet dramatically. Start with time-frames that aren't too long , and you can easily complete without too stress on your body. For instance, you could begin with 15 to 20 minutes, three to 5 times a week to complete your exercise routine. The length and frequency of your exercise can play a significant role in impacting the final results of your workout. It is important to keep focus and determination throughout your work out. In this way, you will increase the strength, endurance, and general fitness levels. This is the best way to go in order to attain the level of fitness you've always wanted.

Refresh, heal, and then continue

When you follow this process by following this method, you will benefit from calisthenics. Whatever type of exercise or everyday activities you're engaged in, it is important to prioritize your break and rest intervals as they are the best times to allow the body to heal and prepare it for the next exercises. When you rest, your muscles also have the chance to recover and create new cells. When you get the right quantity of sleep, you'll soon be able to work out longer at higher levels. When you do your calisthenics you will experience slight tears to the muscle fibers. This is easily repaired and gives an increase in strength and bulkier muscles when you take a break.

Don't overdo your workouts and stay away from rest since this could result in the creation of irreparable damage to the muscle tissues as well as burnout. Also, you are susceptible to injuries when your muscles become stretched without rest. When you create your exercise schedule, be sure to record the days of rest and the proper kinds of rest that are specifically calisthenics-specific. Let's say that the workout that you did just completed was concentrated on the lower regions of your body. To ensure that these parts are rested and not stressed out Your next set of exercises should be focused on another part of your body, such as the chest or arms areas.

Keep track of your workout Sessions

A well-documented recording of your exercise sessions can help in keeping you informed on your progress, determining where changes are required as well as ensuring that the objectives you set to yourself are achieved and, most important, it will motivate you. Recording your exercise sessions is an integral component of the callisthenic workout procedure. Here are some benefits of keeping a record of your workouts;

The physical changes the are experienced by the body during the tour will be noted down

There will be greater accountability and you won't be prone to cheating in your routines.

Based on your fitness records and your current fitness level, you'll find the most effective method that is right for you.

You'll always strive to reach your goals in a realistic manner.

You'll be motivated and the idea of giving up will never ever occur to you.

The Correct Diet Type

Your workouts will require lots of energy. This must always come from the correct source that will supply energy to your muscles at the times it is most essential. The calories are the kinds of energy your body uses during exercise and need replenish the stored energy. There is no one identical bodies, and your energy needs are different than the other person. What you consume in calories are the ones you will have available to you throughout your exercise. Because calisthenics is a very high energy sport the calories you consume will be much more than other exercise kind requires. An additional 300 to 600kcal a day is the optimal energy intake for you.

In order to get the most benefit from your workouts, a gradual procedure should be followed to ensure the proper development. This can be the basis for subsequent exercises, and you must ensure that your goals are aligned with the kind of exercises you plan to perform.

# Chapter 13: Top Exercise Equipment Perfect For Home Workout

Being at home exercising has many advantages. First, you'll cut down on travel time, do not have to wait around so that equipment is ready to use as well as you are able to wear whatever you like while watching your favorite television series. All this and more because you choose to exercise at your home. It is possible to enjoy the same great exercise as you can in any gym. That is, of course, when you have the proper equipment that is suitable within your financial budget.

The following are the best equipment that you can utilize at home. You can begin burning off those fats and building muscles no matter what your budget.

1. Dumbbells

Test your body's strength with dumbbells as opposed to machines. One benefit of using dumbbells is that you are able to work every muscle by using a full range of movements. 3 to 10 pounds are excellent for beginning.

2. Stability Ball

It is among the most beneficial equipments as it is able to be used to perform any workout like hamstring curls, squats, and bench presses. To reduce strain, select the stability ball that is perfect to your size. TIP: Pick an anti-burst ball that doesn't disappear that easily.

3. Jump Rope

The jumping rope is thought to be as one of the most effective forms of exercise that you can do indoors. In addition to its convenience Did you know that you can burn as many as 100 calories in 10 minutes with a moderate pace? The impact can build strength and bone density and agility. It also builds strength and agility.

Keep your eyes on the ball so that you don't to pull your feet off. Tips: Select the one that has an extra weight. This way, you'll lose more calories as well as tone your shoulders and arms.

4. Kettlebell

The kettlebell exercise helps you tone up in just minutes. It encourages natural moves and helps get all muscles working out, leading in increased strength and rapid toning. Tips: Pick a non-slip kettlebell as you'll be working up some sweat. Hot palms and a 10-lb kettlebell could be dangerous.

5. Mat

This piece can take you an enormous step forward with your exercise routine. Make use of a mat for crunches or standing moves. If you are choosing a mat to use pick one with a sticky , grippy surface to help keep your feet and body in place.

6. Treadmill

If you are serious about losing weight should think about purchasing an exercise machine. At least 2.0 HP and a long belt are ideal. It is also possible to choose an exercise machine that has set programs that allow you to accelerate or slow your speed. This will give you a variety of exercise all from the comfort of your home.

7. Stationary Bike

If you're in search of something that is comfortable to use on the knees and in the back without the feeling of an upright bike that is uncomfortable, the stationary bike is the best option. Looking for stationary bikes? Try it out by lifting yourself off the seat as you pedal. This will ensure that it doesn't wobble. The pedal should be soft as many stationary bikes make use of friction, making it difficult to control, giving you a rough ride.

8. Adjustable Bench

To increase the versatility of your workout, purchase an adjustable bench for your home fitness center. This makes it easier to perform decline and incline presses as well as sit-ups, and other abdominal exercises. If you purchase one, it will require a bench that is not very high because it could cause back pain. A little more than 12 inches over the floor while flat is the ideal height. For the best exercise, select the right bench which is adjustable to different places.

# Chapter 14: Diet And Exercise

Many people believe the thinness of a person is a sign to being healthy. However, being overweight can be the same as having a bad life style. Although this is often the case however, recent research has shown that those who are leaner and live a healthy lifestyle are less likely suffer from health issues and are significantly less likely to have a long life. Even if you're thin and don't exercise, it does not mean that you're less healthy than people who are carrying more weight, however, try to exercise regularly.

How important is diet in exercise?

The Dr. Joseph Mercola on his website stated that "exercise and nutrition go hand-in-hand". Indeed, Dr. Mercola claims that having the proper mix of both will "help treat health problems", "lower your risk for diseases" in addition to "help you live a long life full of energy and passion."

If your goal in fitness is weight loss, the routine you follow should be complemented by a healthy diet to allow you to attain your desired goal. If it's getting stronger or having more leaner muscles that you're after the training regimen and diet must work to achieve this. Be aware of what you put in your diet plan will aid you in exercising and should provide you with the daily nutrition that your body needs. A balanced diet is essential!

Fruits and Vegetables, Carbohydrates, and Protein

Carbohydrates -- a lot of people think that if there's a specific kind of food to avoid while losing weight, it's carbs. But, if you're on an intense training schedule you must eat carbohydrates to allow your body to be able to provide a fuel source. Professional athletes and individuals who exercise regularly must eat a lot of carbohydrates. However, if you're the kind of person whose exercise schedule is only

117

a few times a week , or for a short period of time It is recommended to reduce your intake of carbs.

Proteins are essential for those who work out regularly. In contrast to those who lead mostly inactive lifestyles, active people (especially those who are involved in intense training) are advised to consume more protein because it aids in to strengthen and replenish muscles within the body.

Even if you don't exercise eating plenty of vegetables and fruits is essential for every person. It is packed with all the healthy things like fiber and vitamins which are essential to help your body perform. Take in the most fruits and vegetables that you are able to. It's recommended that you consume the most color (green-broccoli or orange-carrots) in the amount you're able in your daily diet.

Vitamins are an effective method to fill in the holes in your diet plan. The book isn't covering all the different kinds of vitamins, however they're a fantastic addition to any exercise and diet program. For instance , taking Vitamin D while strength building can be beneficial as it aids in strengthening muscles and bones.

# Chapter 15: Choosing Suitable Clothing

As discussed in the sections above, exercise in the present is vital to a healthy lifestyle. It helps you shed weight, and strengthen your muscles, allowing them more flexibility. It is advantageous because this type of exercise can be performed both outdoors and indoors, anytime. It also makes you more versatile in your skills and intensity. It's also ideal for those who have not done any kind of exercise before but are looking to start an exercise routine regularly in addition to those who are avid sports enthusiasts.

To ensure that this happens ensure that you're wearing the right clothes. They should be loose, but not too loose Beware of rubber and plastic as they can cause your body temperature rise to dangerous levels. Choose to wear a few lighter layers rather than heavier ones. Also, wear lighter colours during the summer , since they take in heat more slowly.

If you're a beginner or new to exercise, or any other exercise, it's crucial to be at ease. loose fitting clothing allows for free airflow, while tight clothing hinder your movement, rendering your workout ineffective and possibly risking injuries. When you purchase your clothes, rub the fabric to feel what it is like. If the fabric is soft, you'll be more flexible.

If you want to appear trendy and fashionable be sure that the material is comfortable. If you're not able to move in a proper manner you'll lose your energy quickly. Don't spend too much neither. Talk to a fitness instructor or a friend the price your first outfit will cost.

The clothing that you put on the skin must be in a position to absorb moisture. You can wear t-shirts sweatshirts, or tracksuit bottoms, or tights. If you are wearing appropriate clothing your motivation and energy are boosted, making your workout fun.

FOCUS ON EFFORT, NOT DISCOMFORT!

Injuries

Aerobics are a great way to shed weight, increase endurance, and keep your heart healthy however, there could have a negative side. If you exercise not cautiously, you may hurt yourself. Follow these tips to ensure your workout is enjoyable and healthy.

The first step is to think about your clothing. A good pair of workout shoes is also crucial. Aerobics requires a lot of movements. If your footwear is old or the laces come undone easily, you could slide and slide and fall. Check that the rest of your attire isn't overly rigid or heavy, as they could cause heat stress.

Think about your exercise space, particularly if you have a home gym. You should be able to move freely and be sure not to bump into furniture. The equipment should also be serviced frequently, since malfunctioning machinery could be extremely dangerous. The work area that you are working in should be kept clean so as not to be exposed to harmful bacteria or viral infections.

Basic Human Physiology

Happy Healthy Hearts

Everybody knows that working out is beneficial for your body. But, do you comprehend the benefits of cardio and heart health? A lot of people believe that aerobics is the best option to be well and be more effective in all aspects of their lives. Aerobics and heart health are something you should keep an eye on as it will make you feel better and remain fit.

The significance of aerobics in promoting heart health will remain throughout the rest the time. The more you exercise, the more healthy your heart will get.

In terms of the relationship between aerobic exercise and well-being, you're giving your lungs and heart the chance to exercise. They perform harder and more quickly. If you exercise regularly your lungs and heart will get stronger. This means that you'll be able do more aerobic exercise without ever stopping.

It is necessary to build up. If you've not exercised for some time the heart may not be sufficient to handle too many. Make sure to take your time and consult your physician to create an aerobics program which will help you.

The Heart: An Introduction

It is an organ that circulates oxygen-rich blood to the cells of the body. It is essential to our daily life. It beats around 80,000 to 100,000 times a day, and pumps around 2000 gallons of blood into our muscles. The heart beats continuously to ensure that we are alive.

Heart pumps blood to the veins that transport oxygen to the cells of the body. In return towards the heart, the veins carry oxygenated blood to the lung. This is where the blood collects oxygen and then transports this back towards the heart. This helps keep the circulation of blood.

The Heart's Structure

The heart has four chambers within the heart. These are made up of two atriums (singular atrium) and two ventricles. It's pear-shaped and about similar to an average fist. It is located in the lower left part of our body and is protected from the back by the ribs. The heart's muscle , also known as the cardiac muscle is classified as an involuntary muscle because we don't have any control over it.

The Three Layers of the Heart

PERICARDIUM

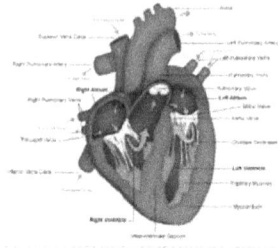

The layer is made up of a hard tissue that covers the heart. It's split to form two layers.

Outer layer - it helps support the heart and keeps it in place by securing to chest cavities.

The inner layer, also known as the epicardium layer is situated on top of the muscle of your heart.

MYOCARDIUM

This layer is made up of the cardiac muscle in and of itself. It is the wall of the four chambers.

ENDOCARDIUM

This layer is composed of a thin connective and endothelial tissue. It is shiny and white, and is a line that runs through the middle layer. Its purpose is to stop blood clots from forming within each of the chambers.

The Circulatory System

The superior vena cana brings deoxygenated circulation to the coronary artery from the higher part of the body, while the inferior vena vena cava draws blood from lower bodies. The vena Cava is comprised of smooth muscle that is elastic and flows to the right atrium. The arteries are elastic, which means they can stand up to the force of pumping.

The right atrium, which is sent by the sinoatrial node on the upper wall of the atrium. Both atria must be contracted simultaneously in order to allow for the continued flow of blood. The blood flows via the tricuspid valve permitting it to flow into the ventricle right. The valves allow blood to flow, and stop the flow.

Now , the blood is flowing into the right ventricle through the AV node located in that lower part of the atrium. This node sends signals through the Bundle of His to the Purkinje fibers to allow the ventricles to expand. The blood is pumped from the right ventricle via the semilunar valve of the pulmonary artery and into the pulmonary artery which is then able to take out the heart. The valves also stop the blood from returning to the ventricle.

The pulmonary artery is the sole arterial route that transports deoxygenated blood. It removes it from the lungs and the heart. The increased blood volume creates the membrane of the lungs to expand because of their cells' sacs. The sacs, known as alveoli, contain capillaries. The blood that was deoxygenated is now passing through these capillaries before being returned to oxygen as we breathe in oxygen. Inhaling and exhale, we release carbon dioxide and return it to the air.

The process that occurs in the lung is called gaseous exchange. It transforms carbon dioxide from the body and the heart back to oxygen. The blood is pumped into the veins that supply the oxygenated blood back to the heart.

The oxygenated blood reaches the right atrium, which causes the walls of the atrium to expand. The blood then flows through the mitral valve or bicuspid valve and into the ventricle left.

| AGE | TARGET RANGE (BEATS/MINUTE) |
|---|---|
| 20-24 | 120-150 |
| 25-29 | 117-146 |
| 30-34 | 114-142 |
| 35-39 | 111-139 |
| 40-44 | 108-135 |
| 45-49 | 105-131 |
| 50-54 | 102-127 |
| 55-59 | 99-123 |
| 60-64 | 96-120 |
| 65-69 | 93-116 |
| 70+ | 90-113 |

The left ventricle is then able to collect the blood, which makes its walls shrink, allowing the blood to flow through the semilunar valve in the aortic to the Aorta.

The aorta, the most important vein that transports oxygenated blood through the heart into other parts of our body. While not all blood flows to the body, however a portion remains behind to provide to the muscle of the heart with oxygen. This allows it to continue moving.

If the body's cells are oxygenated again and blood has taken in carbon dioxide it will send return to the heart through the Vena cava.

How the Heart Beats

The two kinds of heartbeats are:

DIASTOLE - During this kind rhythm, muscles that surround the ventricles loosen which causes pressure to fall. The bicuspid valve opens , allowing the atrias to fill with blood. The valve closes and allows blood flow through the ventricles and cause the ventricles to grow. The blood pressure within the aorta decreases then the valve semi-lunar shuts.

SYSTOLE In this type heartbeat muscle walls of the ventricles begin to contract, which causes the pressure to increase. The tricuspid and bicuspid valves are closed. The aorta pumps blood to the pulmonary arterial, as well as the atria loosen. The left atrium gets blood through the pulmonary vein, as well as the right atrium is supplied by the Vena cava.

Heart Rate

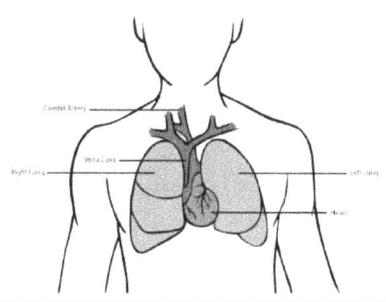

It is crucial to keep track of your heart rate while doing exercises. This will allow you to discern if you're performing the correct exercises and that you are doing them properly. If you're new at fitness your optimal heart rate should be around 50-60 percent of your maximum heart rate. Be sure to do warm-up exercises prior to starting your workout routine. Gradually increasing your heart rate will reduce body fatand lower cholesterol and blood pressure and thus reduce 85 per cent of the calories in your body. If you're an active person who is used to exercising your heart rate target is between 60 and 70 percent that of the maximum rate you can achieve. This will result in faster weight loss and will burn more calories. The optimal heart rate is 70-80 percent.

TABLE TO SHOW TARGET HEART RATES IN BEATS PER MINUTE

When resting 5 litres of blood flow every minute.

(0.07l.x 70 Beat per minute= 4.9l. per minute).

Aerobics Trims the Heart

Through years of studying the effects of heart disease researchers were able to create some incredible results. Through regular exercise, you can shrink an overly large heart. A heart that is smaller means it's a better organ to pump blood. Another study was conducted on people suffering from heart insufficiency. The results revealed that when patients exercised regularly throughout the week, their hearts started to pump more efficiently.

The USA alone, there are approximately five million patients who suffer from heart failure. This causes a large number of patients being hospitalized, which results in expenses to the health system that range from thirty to $30 billion.

If someone has suffered for long-term heart failure These people typically have high blood pressure, which can eventually cause an attack on the heart. The heart gets bigger that is in poor shape, and then becomes too weak to pump blood.

For a long time doctors would refrain from prescribing exercises to patients suffering from heart problems. They gave lots of rest in bed to ease the stress on the heart. Over the last 10 years studies have shown that exercising is beneficial. It helps reduce the signs of heart failure and counteracts the negative adverse effects of hormones. These improvements aid in compensating for the weak points that are created within the heart.

The oxygen added to in the heart when aerobics is taking place triggers chemical changes. The heart now can circulate oxygenated blood throughout the body with greater efficiency. The lung capacity of the body increases and more oxygen can be absorbed into the body. Oxygen helps strengthen the muscle of the heart, so that the body is able to detox more effectively, decreasing the chance of developing illness. This heart activity boosts HDL which eliminates bad cholesterol from blood.

Aerobics may lower blood pressure, so that the heart can do more however, we perform it with more effort, which allows your body to feel more fit and healthy, prevent illness, experience no fatigue, and have better, more precise memory.

Heart and Lungs Work Together

While you're exercising the more blood is flowing to your muscles. The rate will rise by 4 to 5 times that of the resting rate.

The sympathetic nerve stimulates respiratory muscles to boost their rate of breathing. Dietary byproducts (waste) include hydrogen ions, lactic acid and carbon dioxide, stimulate the brainstem's nerve centers to stimulate the muscles. The blood pressure increases with the increase in heartbeat and cardiac output. This opens the channels to the alveoli within the lung. This is sure to boost ventilation and bring more oxygen to the bloodstream to aid in helping muscles to work at their maximum capacity.

# Chapter 16: The Science Behind Physical Fitness

According the Dr. Cheng, if the advantages of exercising can be incorporated into a drug the result would be worth one million dollars. The researchers have been intrigued by the benefits of exercising regularly. Their results are positive. Here are some of the findings.

Boosts the Immune System

A study from 2017 revealed that a moderate 20-minute workout is extremely beneficial to your immune system. The study included 47 healthy participants. Participants were asked to walk or run along a treadmill dependant on their fitness levels. Prior to and following the workout they assessed the levels of an inflammatory marker TNF. They discovered that there was the reduction of 5% in the amount of immune cells producing the marker.

This study suggests that physical activity can improve the immune system by stopping excessive inflammation. The study discovered that exercise can have anti-inflammatory effects. However, they weren't capable of describing the process by which this happens. Inflammation is a normal response by the immune system illnesses and injuries. But, if it's too much, it may cause harm. It can cause discomfort and even harmful consequences.

So, the fact that this study demonstrated that exercise has antiinflammatory properties is an excellent sign. It shows that it can safeguard you from chronic ailments because of moderate inflammatory reactions. This is an exciting result as it indicates that you could never need to buy anti-inflammatory medicines to protect yourself from the risk from a rash of inflammation. Thus it appears that it appears that Dr. Cheng was right when he stated that the benefits of exercise can be worth millions of dollars.

Reduces Cancer Risk

Cancer, in all its varieties, can be a debilitating illness that causes pain to many people across the globe. The treatment for it can be challenging due to the fact that it typically requires surgery that is costly and can have many adverse negative effects. So it is best to avoid the method to combat this condition. The positive aspect is one way to lower the chance of developing cancer is by exercising regularly.

Studies have demonstrated that regular physical exercise is linked to decreases in the risk of colon and breast cancer. A review of various studies found that moderate physical exercise has a more impact on protection than lower intensity activities. The study revealed that people who are physically active women can enjoy an increase of 30% to 40% in the chance of developing colon cancer. Women, in particular are experiencing an average of 20%-30% less the chance of developing breast cancer.

The main conclusion from this review of systematic reviews is that there's solid evidence that exercising can lead to a reduction in the frequency of specific cancers. The authors believe that those who regularly exercise have a lower chance to suffer from colon or breast cancer specifically. Researchers also found that cancer patients active in sports and recreation are less at risk of developing cancer when compared with those who are not as active.

>>>Watch The Video Home Workout System<<<

Prevents Cardiovascular Disease

Generallyspeaking, regular exercise raises you heartbeat, and this is good for overall well-being. Researchers believe that women particularly are less likely of dying from specific illnesses caused by physical inactivity. One of them is heart disease.

Furthermore, research has proven that women and men who exercise regularly are less likely to being afflicted by heart-related ailments.

A case in point is a study that examined the effects exercising in middle age males and women, and followed them over eight years. Researchers discovered that the lower quintiles of physical fitness were linked to an increased risk of dying due to cardiovascular diseases. The top quintiles had an lowered risk of death. The research further has confirmed that the likelihood of suffering from this illness are much lower than previously considered. Recent studies have shown that being active and fit can provide a more than 50% decrease in the likelihood of dying from heart-related ailments. The research also revealed that middle-aged women who were physically inactive had a 52% increase in mortality due to all causes. They do less than an hour of physical activity each week. Researchers also found that women with this condition have an increase of 29% in mortality due to cancer in comparison with their more physically active counterparts.

Decreases Chances of Diabetes

The effects of diabetes can affect your life in a negative manner. In addition to causing pain and pain, it can also stop you from enjoying some of your most loved foods. But, researchers have found that you can shield yourself from the effects of this condition by participating in regular exercise. A study for instance found that resistance and aerobic forms of exercise can be effective in preventing the development of type 2 diabetes. The study included 46 participants who engage in energy-consuming activities.

The study found that exercising regularly reduces the chance of developing Type 2 Diabetes by six percent. They observed that this advantage was most evident for those with a higher BMI. These people are at greater risk of developing diabetes than other people. However, this study proved that in addition to losing weight, exercising increases the odds of becoming a diabetic. A number of studies have confirmed the findings, proving the results are valid.

A study, for instance, that involved 271 male doctors recorded similar results. The study showed that individuals who reported a weekly physical exercise had lower incidence of diabetes type 2. The exercises they performed made them sweat. Researchers explained that participants also have a lower likelihood of suffering from cardiovascular disease.

Improves Bone Health

If you're looking to increase the density of your bones, you have to establish a routine of regularly exercising. Resistance exercise, specifically weight-bearing exercise, has the greatest impacts on bone mineral density. A cross-sectional review of numerous studies showed that resistance exercise increases the density of bone. Thus, those who engage in these types of activities have a greater chance of having stronger bones than those who don't engage in these exercises.

Furthermore the authors found that the kind of sport you participate in affects the calcium mineral count. For instance, those who play sports with low impact generally have lower bone density as compared to athletes who participate in high-impact sports. So, while exercising helps improve bone health, particular exercises have more significant effects more than other exercises. Researchers have also seen similar results from studies that involved young children, adolescents, middle age and even older adults.

Numerous longitudinal studies have studied the impact of exercise on bone health in different categories of people. Researchers suggest that further research is needed, specifically those with more participants. However, the research up to now have demonstrated that there is evidence that physical activity improves bone health. They also decrease the likelihood of suffering from bone-related ailments. Research suggests that weight-bearing and impact exercises allow you to avoid the loss of bone due to the aging process.

# Chapter 17: Nutrition

The second aspect of having an incredible body is the nutritional program we follow. At the start, we have to eliminate "toxic" food and replace them with healthier options that are lower in calories. We will then follow a strict eating plan and use the only method I have found to be efficient intermittent fasting. I've been using this method for the last two years and the results I saw after the first six months were remarkable. I would highly recommend intermittent fasting for all my clients who are elderly to fight the slowing of metabolism we face at the age of 40.

I've never experienced the chest striations and the veins on my shoulders and I am proud to stand with the intermittent fasting side that has spread across the fitness industry and with great reason. I've included the entire guide to getting started on this program as well as a simple nutritional guideline page.

If you're not sure about intermittent fasting, we'll explain briefly, after which we'll go over the fundamentals of nutrition, then we'll be going into the incredible advantages and benefits of intermittent fasting. It permits an eating plan that is not governed by as many limitations, while still encouraging the loss of fat and muscle and making it easier to save time and money.

Intermittent fasting is a diet program that involves deliberately eating a diet for a time, and then consuming the amount of food you like in your food-window. This method is revolutionary and allows certain weight loss within a brief time, and does not limit the types of food you are able to eat. How and why does intermittent fasting is beneficial and what are the benefits and the reason to use this incredible method to lose weight for maximum results quickly and easily? These are the questions we'll address with some helpful tips to ensure that your intermittent fasting is easy and easily without the need to deal with cravings that aren't within your food window.

How does intermittent fasting function? Prior to beginning to learn the fundamental routine of intermittent fasting you must know the way the weight gain and loss are a function from a strictly scientific perspective.

The weight loss strategy is with magic supplements or methods that are founded on the science of the physiognomy. Intermittent fasting is more effective than other strategies or diets but it's all based on the basic logic that people tend to ignore.

The Basics

The importance of nutrition is paramount to any fitness plan. Your body can do incredible things, just consider how your body develops and grows in the beginning of our lives. Our bodies are only the weight of a few pounds. Yet we quickly build stronger muscles, bones strengthen and grow Our entire body adjusts to new demands. To accomplish this however, the body requires specific sources. Humans are omnivores, but we need certain vitamins and minerals that can be found only in vegetables, meat fruits, grains that, in the XXI. century, we are able to supplement with. It is important to remember that supplements cannot rival healthy food in the real world.

The relationship between food intake and weight loss occurs when it comes to our caloric intake. The majority of people are aware of the Kilocalorie and calorie measurement The scientific definition of calorie can be described as "A calory or calorie (archaic) is an measurement of energy. There are many definitions, but they can be classified into two broad categories. One, known as the smaller calorie (symbol Cal) refers to the volume energy required to raise the temperature of a Gram in water 1 degree Celsius at an atmospheric pressure of 1 atmosphere. The other, the larger calories or kilocalorie (symbols: Cal, kcal) and also referred to in the context of the food calorie, and similar terms can be defined as the energy needed to increase temperatures of one kilogram (rather than one kilogram) of liquid by an inch Celsius. It's equivalent to 1000 small calories."

Our bodies require certain calories each day in order to lead a healthy lifestyle. The amount varies from individual to individual, based on factors like gender, height and. There are a variety of formulas to use to calculate our calories, but the most straightforward and most efficient option is to search on the internet to find " calories calculator ", and then fill in an online form. For those who want to do it on their own we suggest using the World Health Organization's equation for 1980.

Formula :

Females Age 3 to 9 years = 22.5 * (Weight in kilograms) + 499 Ages 10-17 years equals 12.2 1 (Weight in kilograms) + 746 Age 18-29 years = 14.7 1.47 (Weight in kilograms) * 496 Age 30-60 years = 8.7 8 (Weight in kilograms) + 829 Age above sixty years equals 10.5 (Weight in kg) (Weight in kilograms) + 596

Males Ages 3-9 years = 22.7 (Weight in kg) + 495 Age 3 to 9 years = 22.7 (Weight in kilograms) + 495 Ages 10-17 years = 17.5 (Weight in kg) (Weight in kilograms) Plus 651 18-29 years = 15.3 (Weight in kg) (Weight in kilograms) Plus 679 30-60 years = 11.6 * (Weight in kilograms) plus 879 above 60 is 13.5 * (Weight in kilograms) + 487

Let's say that you're a woman aged 22. The typical American woman who is over 20 weighs 168.5 pounds and is about 5'3 inches. Based on this data when we incorporate this information into an online calculator of calories in the event that you live an active lifestyle that involves

151

minimal or no physical activity We'll discover that you'll need 1,789 calories per day. this amount can vary depending on the activities you engage in and that's why we suggest using a calculator online to determine precisely how many calories you actually require. This figure shows the number of calories you must consume to keep your weight in check.

It is evident that things will change when you're an older male of 52 seeking to improve their physique. That's why we have included formulas for all ages to help you determine the calories required to consume.

The fundamental principle behind weight loss and gain is very simple. You consume less calories than what you need and you lose weight. you consume more calories than you require and the body weighs more.

We stated that "you lose weight", not fat. In fact, by eating fewer calories than what you need and losing weight, but you also lose muscles. This is the reason why it is suggested to exercise when trying to shed excess fat. Not only does it speed the process however it also helps maintain our muscle massand can help to shed as much fat as is possible while losing less as possible muscle. A second thing to note is that we refer to the word "nutrition", not "diet". The reason is that people who are fit think of eating healthy as to be a way of life, whereas eating a diet is something you can do for a specific duration of time.

In the next article we will discuss the best way to apply these guidelines in order to shed fat, based on your goals and determination. We've said that you can not exercise, but nevertheless lose weight, with much of that being fat. If your aim is to make your abs display, you might want to increase the thickness of your arms for males, or slim your legs and your butts as a woman, in order to appear the best you can this summer, fitness and a stricter diet will be necessary.

It is possible to find out the calories included in each meal at the bottom of the packaging or on the internet. Based on that information and using the kitchen scale you can calculate the number of calories you consumed at each meal. There are numerous applications for tracking calories that you can download to your phone rather than writing it down each meal. We recommend using apps as they make it simpler to track the calories you consume each day and every week.

Before we get into the specific nutrition plans according to how committed you are, let's look at the foods you need to stay clear of if you want to shed some weight. These contain a lot of calories, are low in minerals and vitamins which is why they should be avoided or substituted for low-calorie, healthy alternatives.

Soda, or any other beverage except for coffee, tea, or water is best avoided. We recommend that you drink coffee or tea that is not sweetened with sugar, or with artificial sweeteners like Stevia. Alternatives to these drinks is to choose zero sugar alternatives that are less healthy however they contain very little or no calories.

Pasta - opt for Whole grain noodles or rice noodles.

Pastries are a great source of carbs and calories. Not filling, pastry shouldn't touch your food or your mouth if you're aiming to build the summer body.

Sweets are anything that falls in the category of sweets, desserts or sweets, is likely to be considered to be a threat. There is no sugar in chocolate or candy in the majority of stores, and usually made by Stevia. We will also cover a variety of delicious snacks to enjoy, which won't harm your body.

Fast food is another obvious one, but no hamburgers, fires or tacos, fried chicken or anything else you can find from a drive-through place should be eaten. A majority of the foods you eat must be prepared at home, or, if dining out, you should choose an establishment and not an eatery that serves fast food.

Deep-fried foods are anything that is fried in lots of oil, ranging from fired chickens and French fries. Healthy alternatives include dishes prepared in the oven with a touch of olive oil and sweet potato fires that are cooked by baking.

White bread substitute white bread with whole grain bread or an alternative that is even better than bread slices could be rice cakes.

White rice. You can replace it it with brown rice.

Alcohol : All alcohol must be avoided, if you wish to enjoy drinks with the occasion such as white wine, blonde beers and gin are the tiniest calorific drinks that you can drink.

If you can stop eating these foods, you may shed a few pounds over the shortest amount of time. A friend from high school gained more than 40 pounds in the span of five months through a cessation of sweets, sodas and bread.

Once you have identified the food items that can keep your weight loss There are a few snack options that are quick and easy to consume anytime you have cravings.

• A few nuts ( roughly as much that you are able to fit into one hand)

Shakes with protein ( of the flavor you like)

*Popcorn ( few calories )

* Greek fruit yoghurt, topped with fresh fruit

* Fruits ( not including grapes and pears due to the high amount of sugar they contain )

* Candy that is sugar-free

* Protein bars

* Oatmeal

* Rice cakes topped with orange slices

* Dark chocolate ( 1 to 2 squares )

After providing you with some general guidelines on food items to avoid and those that you should try, we'll go into greater detail on how you can apply this knowledge to shed weight or fat according to the level of commitment you have.

The easiest method

The most basic method of weight loss has one simple requirement to eat less calories than you require. Although there is much debate about what the ideal number is but a good starting point could be between 400- 500 calories less per day. Therefore, if, according to your information, you need to take in 1800 calories and aim to eat only 1300 - 1400.

A kitchen scale is a great way to measure the quantity of food items and calories in them and putting yourself on an energy deficit has been scientifically proven to help you lose weight, according to how your body functions. In this way, however, you'll be losing weight and muscles.

We're not going to complicate matters for our readers, we suggest cutting out the food items we've listed to avoid and changing to healthier alternatives along with tracking calories in order to reach the caloric deficit of 400 to 500 kcal, you'll be in good shape. We do suggest following the more difficult route by exercising regularly and eating a range of foods that we'll outline in the following section, in order to unlock that body you've always dreamed of.

As we mentioned at this article, the best method to shed weight and create a more healthy body is to combine nutrition and exercising. First that you eat healthy foods. Eliminate all the food items listed in this category, and concentrate on eating premium products. Utilizing your kitchen scale, take measurements of your meals and calculate the caloric content.

When we get into nutrition, you'll need to realize that food is composed of three main macro-nutrients. They are carbohydrates, fats and proteins. The most crucial of these three, in terms of fitness perspective is protein. Protein is essential to build and maintain muscle and typically, protein-rich food items are also less in calories.

The foundation of any program to lose weight:

- A slight caloric deficit ( aprox. 200 kcal )

- Protein-rich foods

Foods of high quality

- A large amount of veggies

- Water ( Hydration )

A few helpful tips and tricks are listed at the bottom of this section

As we try to make this program as simple as we can for you, we're going to give you specific recipes for every breakfast of the week. It is expected that you will consume 3 main meals, and two snacks.

Breakfast: Protein, Carbohydrate, Fruit

Lunch: Protein, Carbohydrate, Fruit or Vegetable

Dinner: Protein, Carbohydrate, Vegetable

Snack 1: Fruit

Snack 2 Snack 2: A snack on the list below.

Protein ideas:

1. Chicken breast

2. Chicken drumstick

3. Tuna

4. Lean beef

5. Lean pork

6. Cottage cheese

7. Eggs ( superfood )

8. Protein powder made from Whey

9. DIY shake ( we'll come back to this )

Carbohydrates ideas:

1. Brown rice

2. Wholegrain bread

3. Sweet potato

4. Oatmeal

5. Beans

Fruit suggestions You can eat nearly any fruit you want but we suggest avoid plums and grapes for fruit the serving size should be 1 portion. 1 banana, 1 orange, 1 apple, etc.

Vegetables: You should avoid regular potatoes. Other aside, you may add other vegetables in any amount.

Snacks:

1. A handful of nuts

2. 2 rice cakes topped with a the thin layer of honey, cinnamon

3. Greek yogurt with fresh strawberries

4. Two teaspoons peanut butter

5. Two squares dark chocolate

6. Two handfuls of popcorn

7. 5 low calorie biscuits

These are your primary ingredients. Since we don't want overcomplicating things for you. Below is an illustration of how to portion your meals. The majority of your plate should include vegetables A quarter should be filled with protein and the other quarter should be filled with carbohydrates.

This is basically all the information you should be aware of about nutrition to lose fat. We'll also discuss some of the strategies and tips that we've found to be extremely useful. remember that results can't be obtained by just doing some big things. it's also the smaller aspects that can add up.

Tips and Tricks

* Cinnamon can help burn fat. Consuming just 1-2 teaspoons of it daily will assist you in burning off fat, but you shouldn't consume it on its own, but you can incorporate it into your food and drink. One teaspoon of cinnamon in your morning cup of coffee, or 1 in your Greek yogurt, and you're well on your way to a healthier lifestyle.

Consuming a banana or any other fruit prior to training will boost your energy levels dramatically.

* Drinking 3L of fluids every day. It may sound like a lot when you have set goals for yourself, such as drinking a bottle of 1L during your workout, drinking 1L from the morning until noon, and one additional liter distributed throughout the day, it's not that difficult.

Sleeping in early can help reduce the risk of cravings that come late at night.

* Drink a glass water prior to every meal and before you go to bed.

Intermittent Fasting

After you've gained fundamental knowledge about the way our body's weight loss or gain systems work, it's time to pose the question "So how and why does intermittent fasting work?"

Intermittent fasting offers greater flexibility in your diet since it's not as strict than the traditional diet that we have discussed above, and gives the possibility to eat on your favourite foods during your meal time. It's just not the time to dispel the most popular myth about intermittent fasting. The truth is that it's the effective fasting that makes the difference.

There are three main components to the fasting plan:

Alternate day fasting 24/24 1:10

165

This type of fasting is the most difficult type to follow because it requires all day without eating and then gives you a full day of eating without restriction. This process repeats as long as you're able to continue to do it, however the biggest drawback is the need to manage your appetite throughout the day, which could make the daily chores difficult due to a lack of energy. This is especially true for those who exercise. You may have read the section on the importance of nutrition and weight loss exercise is a major factor in any goal to shape your body as well as working out with no food intake for a whole day is a challenge and can even trigger catabolism, a procedure of breaking up muscle fibres to create energy. Of course, there's the possibility of exercising on the times when you aren't restricted to fasting but it could cause inconsistency during training, particularly when you train five times per week.

Day 1 Day 2 Day 3 Day 4 Day 5 Day 6 Day 7

Day 8 Day 9 Day 10 Day 11 Day 12 Day 13 Day 14

Day 15 Day 16 Day 17 Day 18 Day 19 Day 20 Day 21

Day 22 Day 23 Day 24 Day 25 Day 26 Day 27 Day 28

Day 29 Day 30 Day 31

Fasting Eating

5 : 2 Fasting

The other fasting plan will make things a little lighter, but is the most ineffective for weight loss. The principle is five days of normal eating and two days of fasting. This in reality isn't that significant.

Day 1 Day 2 Day 3 Day 4 Day 5 Day 6 Day 7

Fasting Eating

Although it is still necessary to go two full day without food, five remaining days are sufficient to make up for the deficit in calories created during those two days.

The 16:8 intermittent fasting ratio

The most likely fasting method as it relates to difficulty and efficiency is that it focuses on fasting for one day instead of over months or weeks. This means that instead of having full days of fasting and full days of eating, it has the benefit of eating daily, and still being on a daily fast. The basic structure of this method is 16 hours fasting and 8 eating.

In terms of difficulties, the 16 : 8 method is the most effective because you don't need to endure days without food, but it's the simplest of the difficult one. It's not likely that intermittent fasting is easy to accomplish for everyone. That's why we'll take a the time to look at some of the techniques and tricks to follow while fasting to help people to adhere to this technique of fasting to achieve the weight loss you want to achieve.

In terms of efficiency, this program permits daily training, as during the 8-hour eating window, you have the opportunity to replenish your energy levels and then get moving at the gym, and the 16 hour fasting interval can be enough to trigger the weight loss mechanisms.

Getting started

If you are the first to begin intermittent fasting, it is recommended to finish your last meal of the day at 20:00. so that your fasting schedule will begin at a point that makes it the most comfortable to manage. You won't be able to eat until 12 noon the next day, which is at noon. Between 12:00 and 20:00, you're in your eating window, and that's the time frame for eating the entire meals you consume that day.

In the beginning, it may be difficult to wake up until 12 noon without eating a single bite. the only food items you're allowed to drink are tea, water as well as black coffee of course, without sweeteners or sugar. We recommend black coffee because milk contains calories and is a part of food items, thus ending your speed.

Another issue with fasting is having cravings at 20:00 since you're no longer in the eating window which is the most frequent time for snacking.

Before we dive into the research that underlies Intermittent Fasting, let's go through some suggestions for making it as simple as it is to fast and not feel the desire to consume food.

The primary reason for the idea behind Intermittent Fasting work, is to give you a feeling of fullness for a longer time. There are some nutrients that help in this and there are a some small tips to avoid having cravings.

#1. Sleep well

One of the major reasons teens and young adults tend to be obese or, perhaps more fat than older generations is the insufficient sleep. It is widely considered by researchers to be connected with the levels of ghrelin as well as leptin hormones. Insufficient sleep raises the levels of ghrelin which is the hormone responsible for feeling of hunger. It also helps in diminuting leptin, the hormone that causes the sensation of being full.

Combining these steps significantly affects the effectiveness of any program to lose weight, or the control of binge eating Therefore, tonight you may want to you should skip a couple of episodes of your preferred Netflix program, then then end the chat earlier, since the recommended duration of sleep is 8 hours to reduce the cravings and reduce binge eating.

Research has concluded that a sleep duration of less than 8 hours per night is associated with a heavier body.

In all honesty that by sleeping earlier, you eliminate the possibility of eating more and you will spend 8 to 10 hours during your 16 hour fasting duration sleeping.

#2. Increase protein intake

Protein and fiber have been scientifically proven to assist with weight loss and related cravings So let's take a look at each one in isolation.

Protein can be described as the single most valuable nutritional element for those who train, and with good reason. It's the most important nutrient linked with muscle development, increased metabolism, and encouraging fullness. The study that saw their participants boost their intake of protein by 15 percent, not only demonstrated a reduction in body weight and mass of fat, however, they also had decreased daily intake of calories at an average of 444 calories.

A few common protein-rich food items include eggs as well as tuna, chicken breasts Protein shakes, fish, and protein shakes All of them are excellent for weight loss programs of any kind.

#3. Consuming more fiber

Fiber is absorbed slowly by your digestive tract which makes you feel full for a longer period of time. It is pure magic in terms of reducing cravings, reducing binge eating and calories consumed, since it can make us feel fuller and for a longer time. Numerous studies support this. The most appealing aspect of fiber is how affordable it is. Fruits and vegetables, whole grains and all whole grains are filled with fiber, however the most beneficial choice for this food that is a star is oatmeal. Oatmeal is incredibly cheap and can be made in many different methods, based on your preference. from protein oats, to fruit oats. It's totally your choice.

#4. Drink more water

Hydrating your body is perhaps the easiest and most efficient method to combat the cravings and hunger. There are a variety of factors at play in this assertion The first is the physical part when you consume greater amounts of water you consume less. When you fill your stomach by drinking water, less space is available for food and it is proven every time. If you'd like to verify this for yourself, prior to your next meal drink 500ml of water. Then determine how much you eat, in comparison to what you would normally eat.

Studies have shown that an increase in consumption of water can lead to weight loss and decreased cravings. One study, carried out on 30 adults found that when they were given 500ml of drinking water prior to eating the food, they ate 13% less calories than those who didn't drink any water.

The athletes who are active drink more water than average people, due to the potential advantages to their body and performance. Another study has shown that drinking water can be associated with boosting the metabolism of your body, which, together with its positive impact could be an important part of the process that suppresses hunger.

What exactly is intermittent fasting? work?

As nutritional and medical experts will tell you that weight loss does not occur because of the fasting process itself or any of the undergoing effects that happen during fasting. The cause is much more straightforward.

The reason people gain weight during fastingeven though they consume normal meals, without limitations, is in the eating time itself. It is difficult to consume more calories than you requirements, when you need to consume them within 8 hours.

Research has shown that people who were on intermittent fasting were able to consume less calories than they needed for the day and a continuous caloric deficit developed. A caloric deficit leads to weight loss in any way, but is more difficult to attain if one is allowed to consume food all day long.

In the end, Intermittent Fasting relies on teaching its adherents to eat within an 8-hour time frame In this scenario it becomes highly likely that they will not eat in excess of calories and instead, they'll be in deficit. Added that the majority of people will maintain a healthy diet when fasting. The results are virtually certain.

However, there is a caveat that, even if you adhere to intermittent fasting and during the 8-hour period, you consume a lot of calorific foods, and then find yourself eating more than the caloric requirement the weight gain will begin be evident. The likelihood of this scenario happening is very minimal, so you attempt to limit yourself to eating healthier food choices, while eating your favourite treats in a reasonable amount you're all set!

# Chapter 18: Using Intensity Techniques To Unlock Your Full Potential

If you now understand the mechanism behind muscle growth, you can begin to apply this knowledge to your training at home. The most important thing is to understand that in order to build microtears. You need to cause metabolic stress, and challenge your body with weights that are increasing. It is important to make sure you are getting enough sleep and protein to ensure the body is able to build back up.

Here's the place where difference is apparent in a variety of home-based workouts. Because if you're lifting a weight, making it curl ten times, and then putting it back down in a row, you're not really doing any work.

You're using a fiber that's fast and a slow twitch fiber to move a heavy object 10 times. You're creating several metabolites and possibly causing some tears, but not enough for an increase in speed.

It is important to train as the bodybuilder.

What exactly does this mean? It means that you must create the maximum amount of stress and damage to your muscles, and test yourself. This is in turn exploring the boundaries and being imaginative.

The Weider Intensity Principles

The 70s are frequently described as the "golden period of bodybuilding. In the 70s, there were numerous big names raising the profile of the sport. These included Arnold Schwarzenegger, Franco Columbu, Lou Ferrigno, Frank Zane, Sergio Oliva etc.

Much of this acclaim could be due to the media maverick Joe Weider, who observed the training of these bodybuidlers and studied their methods used to stimulate growth. He codified these methods to form the Weider Principles that included things like supersets, burns reps and so on. If you've ever had the opportunity to train with a fitness trainer, you've likely seen some of these methods!

In the beginning, Joe neither the bodybuilders he studied from were not aware of how to apply these techniques. Instead, they learned by paying attention to their bodies, and then beginning to notice the indicators that a workout was delivering. As it turns out that all of these methods caused tears in muscles or producing pump. We can pick a few and incorporate them into our own home workouts to make them more efficient.

Particularly I'm studying one of these methods and then another variation of it. This will transform how you train for a lifetime.

Seriously.

What's the method I'm discussing? It's called The Drop Set. Drop sets are a exercise that starts with a large weight that you could lift for around 8-12 reps. Then you do your sets as usual until you fail.

When you've reached a point at which you are unable to lift the weight any more You can simply lower it a bit and keep going.

Let's suppose you're doing curls at the gym. It could be a method known as 'running the rack' that is, you'll go up and down the rack until you get to the lowest weight. It is possible to start with 15kg each hand and do 6-8 repetitions. You could then take them off, and then select 12kg weights, and complete 5 reps. After that, you'll set them down, then pick up 10kg, and complete 6 reps. Then, put them down take 8kg, then do 5 reps. Finally, you'll finish with 4kg, and only do 4 reps prior to collapsing.

This is a set. This means that you must repeat this process three times.

Why is this effective? It's simple: it's causing greatest amount of muscle damage and is increasing the size of the muscle by metabolic waste.

At the beginning in the gym, you'll be lifting a significant weight, and you'll do 6-8 repetitions. That's as many reps as you can manage and you're required to activate a significant amount of muscle fibers, particularly those with fast twitch muscles that can exhaust rapidly. When the fast twitch muscle fibers have been exhausted and torn and strained, your slower twitch muscle will be activated to help. At some point, you'll be unable to have enough strength together to sustain the effort until you're unable to carry the weight any longer. At the same time you'll make the switch from the glycolytic system which lets you extend your.

However, you're not stopping in the middle of a failing! You're taking on a heavier weight and lifting it. This allows you to activate your slow twitch fibers continually and continue to wear out the remaining fast twitch fibers which remain active, causing additional microtears. While doing this you'll be able to achieve an extended period of tension, as you'll soon be doing 20 reps. The muscles begin to get filled with an acid called lactic, which causes the sensation of burning as a result of glycogen's energy system.

Then you end up failing, but you then drop the weight, and keep going - completely relying on slow twitch muscle fibers and beginning to break these too, causing major muscle injury.

It eventually gets to the point that even 5kg isn't enough to handle, and at that point you've done the most damage, which can lead to the highest growth for all kinds of. This isn't any different than simply doing 10 repetitions of a workout you're able to comfortably do!

Applying This Method at Home

It's not easy to accomplish at home by yourself unless you own several equipment and a rack that you can slide down. It's expensive, occupies space, and is generally difficult (though it is possible to make use of a machine for resistance! ).

If we want to take a look, let's examine another (and more effective) alternative. The alternative is the mechanical dropping set'. It's going to be the ULTIMATE instrument to break down your muscles as well as stimulating growth. the majority of people don't realize how effective this method is.

# Conclusion

In the preceding chapters, you've learned a lot about the training exercises using resistance bands. Remember that you are able to perform these exercises at the ease at home. The purpose of using resistance bands is that you can boost the intensity of your exercises. Many people aren't at ease with visiting the fitness center or creating their own exercise station. Make the most of the flexibility and access to your resistance bands.

www.ingramcontent.com/pod-product-compliance
Lightning Source LLC
Chambersburg PA
CBHW060329030426
42336CB00011B/1259